Pharmacy Foundation
Assessment Questions 1

Pharmacy Foundation Assessment Questions 1

Sonia Kauser, MPharm, PGDip Hosp. Pharmacy, PGDip Advanced Practice, Independent Prescriber (Series Managing Editor)
Advanced Clinical Pharmacist Practitioner
Lecturer in Pharmacy Practice / Assistant Professor Physician Associates

Nadia Bukhari, BPharm, FRPharmS, FHEA, Associate Professor, Pharmacy Practice, UCL (Series Editor)

Habib Shah, MPharm, MRPharmS, Independent Prescriber (Contributor)
Calderdale & Huddersfield NHS Foundation Trust Clinical Pharmacist
PCN Trainee Pharmacist Programme Co-lead
Primary Healthcare Development Exams & Calculations lead
Senior PCN Clinical Pharmacist
Trainee Pharmacist Designated Supervisor

Shaheen Razzaq MPharm, PGCert Advanced Clinical Skills and Emergency Medicine, Independent Prescriber (Contributor)
Advanced Clinical Pharmacist Practitioner.

Eleanor Barnes, MPharm, MRPharmS, PGClinDipAdvPrac, Independent Prescriber (Contributor)
Lead Clinical Pharmacist
Contributor for the West Yorkshire Primary Care Workforce & Training Hub
Sessional OSCE Assessor, University of Bradford

Farah Khan, MPharm, PGDipAdvPract, Independent Prescriber (Contributor)
Advanced Clinical Pharmacist Practitioner

Published by the Pharmaceutical Press
66-68 East Smithfield, London E1W 1AW

(**PP**) is a trade mark of Pharmaceutical Press. Pharmaceutical Press is the publishing division of the Royal Pharmaceutical Society

First published 2023

Printed in Great Britain by TJ Books

ISBN 978 0 85711 450 1

A catalogue record for this book is available from the British Library.

Disclaimer
The views expressed in this book are solely those of the author and do not necessarily reflect the views or policies of the Royal Pharmaceutical Society. This book does NOT guarantee success in the registration exam but can be used as an aid for revision.

Dedicated to Huzaifa and Zaydan

Contents

Preface

Welcome to the foundaton assessment question book. The content has been devised by practicing pharmacists to try and provide practical hints and tips for future pharmacy practice as well as preparation for the pre-registration assessment.

The chapters have been divided according to the current registration weighting (high, medium and low). There are a mixture of both single best answers and extended matching questions. We have also included calculations and reference insert questions. We have tried to create interactive content including images and cased based discussions to help facilitate learning.

Examination Format

The topics that will be covered in the assessment are set out in the registration assessment framework available on the GPhC website.

There are two parts to the assessment:

Part one consists of 40 calculation questions and you have 2 hours to complete these using a calculator.

Part two consists of 120 questions: 90 single best answer questions and 30 extended matching questions. You have 2.5 hours to complete these without the use of a calculator.

Reference sources are provided for both parts and examples are:
- BNF extracts
- Summary of product characteristics
- Diagrams and images
- Medication charts

Part one: Calculations

Each assessment will likely include one calculation from each of the following:

- doses and dose regimens
- dosage and unit conversions
- estimations of kidney function
- displacement volumes and values
- concentrations (e.g. expressed as w/v, % or 1 in x)
- dilutions
- molecular weight
- using provided formulae
- infusion rates
- pharmacokinetics
- health economics
- quantities to supply

These are free text pharmaceutical calculations. The use of calculators is permitted when tackling these questions. The GPhC will provide candidates with calculators for the purpose of the assessment.

For example:
Mrs D is a 75-year-old woman who has just been admitted to your respiratory ward with an exacerbation of asthma. On admission she was weighed at 97 kg and states her height as 5 feet 3 inches. When taking her history, you find she quit smoking 10 years ago and is on the following medicines:

- Fostair 100/6 two puffs BD
- Budesonide 4 mg PO OM
- Phyllocontin Continus (aminophylline) 225-mg tablets, two tablets BD MDU
- Salbutamol 2.5 mg nebulised QDS PRN
- Salbutamol 100-mcg CFC-free inhaler 2–6 puffs QDS PRN via an aerochamber (blue)

How much aminophylline should Mrs D receive over the next 24 hours? Give your answer to the nearest whole number.

Part two: Multiple choice questions with extracts

Some questions in part 2 will require calculations. Questions in part two that relate to clinical care are linked to key therapeutic areas. An individual question may link to multiple therapeutic areas.

Therapeutic area	Weighting
Cardiovascular system	High
Nervous system	High
Endocrine system	High
Infection	High
Genito-urinary tract system	Medium
Gastro-intestinal system	Medium
Respiratory system	Medium
Immune system and malignant disease	Medium
Blood and nutrition	Medium
Musculoskeletal system	Low
Eye	Low
Ear, nose, and oropharynx	Low
Skin	Low
Vaccines	Low
Anaesthesia	Low

Single best answer questions (SBAs)

Each of the questions or statements in this section is followed by five suggested answers. Select the best answer in each situation.

For example:

A patient on your ward has been admitted with a gastric ulcer, which is currently being treated. She has a history of arthritis and cardiac problems. Which of her drugs is most likely to have caused the gastric ulcer?

☐ A Paracetamol
☐ B Naproxen
☐ C Furosemide
☐ D Propranolol
☐ E Codeine phosphate

Extended matching questions (EMQs)

Extended matching questions consist of lettered options followed by a list of numbered problems/questions. For each numbered problem/question, select the one lettered option that most closely answers the question. You can use the lettered options once, more than once or not at all.

For example:
Antidepressants

- ☐ **A** Amitriptyline
- ☐ **B** Citalopram
- ☐ **C** Duloxetine
- ☐ **D** Flupentixol
- ☐ **E** Mirtazapine
- ☐ **F** Moclobemide
- ☐ **G** St John's wort
- ☐ **H** Venlafaxine

For questions 1–4

For the patients described, select the single most likely antidepressant from the list above. Each option may be used once, more than once or not at all.

1. Miss K is a 32-year-old woman on your ward who has a long-standing history of depression related to her chronic illness. She has tried antidepressants in the past but stopped them when she felt better. The medical team tell you that she returns to hospital periodically with relapsed symptoms because she stops taking her medicines. They want to treat her depression but the agent they suggest would not be suitable for Miss K, considering her non-adherence.

2. One of the new GPs in the surgery across the road calls you for some advice. He has a patient with him, Mr B, who is 28 years old and has agreed to try an antidepressant medicine. Mr B is otherwise fit and healthy, but the GP would like your advice on what to prescribe for this new diagnosis of moderate depression.

3. Three months later you get another call from the GP about Mr B, who has not responded well to the initial antidepressants and may be experiencing

a number of side-effects. They want to switch him on to a different agent quickly, if not immediately. You inform the GP that one of the drugs he asked about cannot be started immediately.

4. Mrs C has just been admitted on to your emergency admissions unit after being referred directly from her GP, whom she went to see about her headache. On admission she also complains of palpitations and her BP is 205/100 mmHg. On taking her history you note she is Japanese and still eats a traditional diet, leading you to suspect her antidepressant medicine may have precipitated this condition.

High-risk drugs

Each assessment is likely to include at least one question on each of the following drugs or drug groups:

- antibiotics
- anticoagulants
- antihypertensives
- chemotherapy
- insulins
- antidiabetic drugs
- drugs with a narrow therapeutic index
- non-steroidal anti-inflammatory drugs
- methotrexate
- opiates
- parenteral drugs
- valproate

Paediatrics

Around 20% of questions in the assessment will relate to paediatric patients.

Additional resources

Additional resources are provided for up to 25% of questions in part one and part two of the registration assessment. Examples of additional resources include photographs and dosing information.

Key hints and tips collated from previous students and current pharmacists:

1. Use the registration assessment framework to revise, plan and prepare for the topics that will be examined
2. Prepare yourself with the current structure of the exam (both part 1 and part 2)
3. Map your revision to the registration assessment framework
4. Practice answering questions using online methods
5. Remain as calm as possible throughout the assessment
6. Follow instinct/intuition when rationalising the answer
7. Ensure patient care is always prioritised
8. Practice calculations as often as possible
9. Practice SPC inset questions
10. Prepare and practice questions under timed conditions
11. Work with your peers with case based discussions
12. Use the BNF and current guidance to help support revision
13. Practice as many questions/scenarios as possible
14. Liaise with your tutor for revision and support
15. Practice using online questions to help mimic the real sitting (also practice using online whiteboards)
16. Practice, practice, practice!

Good luck with the registration assessment.

Acknowledgements

With sincere thanks to everyone who has made this book happen, especially the contributors and the PhP team.

About the authors

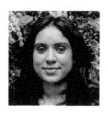

Sonia Kauser, MPharm, PGDip Hosp. Pharmacy, PGDip Advanced Practice, Independent Prescriber

Sonia Kauser is currently an Assistant Professor at the University of Bradford, an Advanced Clinical Practitioner (ACP) in primary care, a director of a primary care service provider and a Primary Care Educator for Health Education England (HEE). She began her career as a pre-registration pharmacy student at Bradford Teaching Hospitals NHS Foundation Trust and then continued her role as a hospital pharmacist. She undertook training in various specialist rotations including paediatrics, oncology, psychiatry, general medicine, surgery, anticoagulation, cardiovascular and respiratory. She was able to pursue a postgraduate diploma in Clinical Hospital Pharmacy at the University of Bradford. Sonia then transferred her skills to primary care in which she began the role of a Clinical GP Pharmacist (based in Yorkshire). This role enabled her to pursue Level 7 Independent Prescribing and her area of specialism was initially anticoagulation. This role has now developed and she undertakes various tasks including working as a senior clinical pharmacist. Sonia then decided to develop her skills and attained a postgraduate diploma in Advanced Practice – Clinical Practitioner, which allows her to manage minor ailment patients within a primary care or urgent care setting. This role allows her to work and support other health care professionals (such as GPs and nurses) by triaging patients and ensuring they are signposted to the correct services. This experience in primary care has allowed her to be part of national pilots for extended access/out of hours schemes.

Sonia has also worked in the following areas: lecturer in pharmacy practice at the University of Manchester, guest speaker for the Royal Pharmaceutical Society, urgent care, out of hours (walk-in centre), GSK (training of pharmaceutical reps), community pharmacy and acute ward pharmacist at Leeds Teaching Hospital.

Sonia enjoys keeping active and reading and shopping in her spare time. Her most recent publications includes contributing for the pharmaceutical oxford press, release of PRAQ 4 (a study book for pre-registration pharmacy students) and an article in the Prescriber Journal which describes the use of clinical information systems to improve practice within primary care.

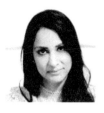 **Nadia Bukhari, BPharm, FRPharmS, FHEA, Associate Professor, Pharmacy Practice, UCL**
Nadia Bukhari is a Principal Teaching Fellow for Pharmacy Practice at UCL. Her interest in writing emerged in her first year of working in academia. Seventeen years on, Nadia has authored ten titles with the Pharmaceutical Press.

She is the Chair for the National RPS Pre-registration Conferences. She developed the extremely popular and over-subscribed conference, when it first started in 2012. Nadia's outreach is wide. She has access to many young pharmacists and is accessible to them through many of her networks. In particular, via her role as an educator for pharmacy undergraduates to her position as Chair for the Royal Pharmaceutical Society national conferences, Nadia directly interacts with almost every trainee pharmacist in England. Her social media presence globalises this interaction on a huge scale.

She has a proven track record within the pharmacy profession and is the UCL Global Pharmacy Ambassador. As well as having a well-known reputation within the pharmacy profession in the U.K, Nadia has also built a global reputation for herself in countries such as Pakistan, UAE, Oman, Poland, Greece, Brazil, Portugal, Italy and Belgium where she has advocated the role of the pharmacist in the U.K.

Nadia has been recognised for her outstanding contributions to the profession by the pharmacy professional body, The Royal Pharmaceutical Society and is the youngest female and youngest Asian to be awarded the status of Fellow of the Royal Pharmaceutical Society. She is the first Muslim woman to have been elected onto the National Pharmacy Board for England, which sets the strategy for the profession and influences on a government level.

Importantly, Nadia uses her platform to be a vocal and prominent advocate for women's rights and is an ambassador and on the Board of Trustees for Pakistan Alliance for Girls Education (PAGE); a charity organisation supported by the government of Pakistan which promotes gender equality in education. In this advocacy role she is currently involved in a huge national project to get more girls going to school in Pakistan. In addition, she has launched the National Alliance for Women in Pharmacy in Pakistan to promote gender equity nationally for female pharmacists.

Following this, Nadia has been appointed as the Global Lead for Gender Equity at the Workforce Development hub for the International Pharmaceutical Federation (FIP).

Leadership in Pharmacy is Nadia's research area of interest and is currently in her final year of study for her PhD.

Nadia is a Fellow of the Higher Education Academy. Nadia is very conscientious and strives to be the best she can be. Teaching and training undergraduates and pharmacists has always been a passion and a drive for Nadia. She always looks for avenues on how to excel her teaching and improve the practice of pharmacy globally.

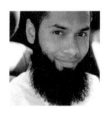

Habib Shah, MPharm, MRPharmS, Independent Prescriber

Habib Shah graduated from the University of Bradford in 2018 with a Master of Pharmacy. He completed his pre-registration placement in a busy community pharmacy located within a medical centre. Due to his exposure within the medical centre, upon qualification, he worked as a practice-based pharmacist implementing policies to improve patient safety. In 2019, he joined Calderdale & Huddersfield NHS Foundation Trust as a clinical pharmacist working across several specialties. Within his role at the Trust, he is currently involved in a pharmacy-led discharge service pilot, which has significantly improved the speed and quality of discharges. Habib is involved in creating & teaching clinical topics to trainee pharmacists at the University of Bradford, within his role as the exam & calculations lead for Pharmacy Foundations, a training provider that provides support to trainee pharmacists. In 2020, he started the role as a PCN pharmacist and was appointed to senior pharmacist and the trainee pharmacist programme co-lead for the PCN in 2022. Habib qualified as an independent prescriber at the University of Bradford in 2021, utilising this skill across primary and secondary care. Habib can be described as a portfolio pharmacist working simultaneously across community pharmacy, general practice, and hospital. His exposure to a variety of settings as an early career's pharmacist placed him in an ideal position to be a designated supervisor to the GP trainee pharmacists working within his PCN. He is also a member of the Yorkshire & Humber trainee pharmacist advisory group. Habib is undertaking a primary care pharmacy education pathway commissioned by HEE, he also hopes to complete an MSc in Advanced Clinical Practice soon.

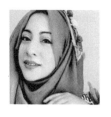

Shaheen Razzaq MPharm, PGCert Advanced Clinical Skills and Emergency Medicine, Independent Prescriber
Shaheen is currently working as the Clinical Lead of Pharmacists in general practice alongside her role as a practice pharmacist in primary care. Her pharmacy journey started in community pharmacy where she took up a management position early on in her career, she continued to want to progress in her role and therefore started the prescribing course which lead her to the world of primary care. She has currently been working in primary care for 7 years and has explored the different areas including urgent care, general practice and out of hours services. She found herself orienting towards general practice and in committing to this journey is now a Clinical Lead overseeing and managing 7 Pharmacists whilst working alongside the clinical lead of other departments to ensure safety and efficiency in patient care. Her greatest goal is to ensure that patient safety is at the forefront of her whole practice and strives towards improving and finding ways to ensure she is constantly developing herself in this area.

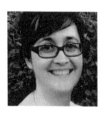

Eleanor Barnes, MPharm, MRPharmS, PGClinDipAdvPrac, Independent Prescriber
Eleanor currently works as a Lead Clinical Pharmacist for a 17-practice GP Federation in Bradford. Her career started in community pharmacy as a Saturday Assistant when she was 15 and shifted to primary care 18 months after she qualified as a pharmacist in 2006. She has spent the second half of her career working in a variety of roles in primary care across West Yorkshire. Eleanor likes to get involved in opportunities in education and training to instil a similar love of primary care pharmacy in those at the very beginning of their careers, and is forging strong links between the University of Bradford, HEE, the local acute trusts and community pharmacies to provide tri-partite training opportunities for undergraduate and post-graduate pharmacists and pharmacy technicians.

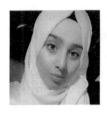 **Farah Khan, MPharm, PGDipAdvPract, Independent Prescriber**

Farah Khan started her MPharm degree at the University of Bradford in 2012, which was the first year that the teaching style had been changed to Team-based Learning (TBL) and this experience hugely helped shape the Pharmacist she is today. Farah is currently working as an Advanced Clincal Practitioner (ACP) at the Caritas Group Practice in Halifax where she plans to continue to develop her skills in broader minor and major ailments and other specialist areas such as dermatology.

She began her journey as a pre-registration pharmacy student in an independent community pharmacy by the name of Harden Pharmacy under the supervision of experienced and super knowledgable pharmacists, and much of her passion to develop and further study was ignited here. Her second pre-registration placement was at a flagship store with Boots which, after working with such a hard-working and inspirational pre-reg tutor, she was influenced to continue working for Boots and develop her skills. After qualifying in 2017, and with further specialised training, she was chosen to become a travel vaccine and services pharmacist for the local flagship stores in the West Yorkshire area. She then moved on to a managerial role in a busy store with Rowlands Pharmacy that was next door to a few GP surgeries. With this she was able to build relations and work closely with different prescribers. It was here that she had decided to pursue a career in Primary Care.

Farah then completed her Independent Prescribers course at the University of Huddersfield, with a specialist interest in diabetes to help tackle, what is now a major public health concern. During and after this time, she worked with companies such as Prescribing Support Services and Prescribing Care Direct (PCD) respectively, to support a variety of Primary Care Networks (PCNs). She has received many opportunities and built amazing connections with other pharmacists, prescribers, practitioners and surgeries via working with Prescribing Care Direct which has provided a great support network for difficult situations in GP practice. This role comprised of training up and tutoring other pharmacists to become a valuable member of the team to help amend and make protocols to manage workload during the Covid-19 pandemic. During this time, she has also managed to successfully complete the Primary Care Pharmacy Education pathway over an 18-month period, to further enhance her clinical and primary care knowledge.

Alongside working with PCD and various PCNs, Farah decided to train as an Advanced Clinical Practitioner with the University of Bradford. Her training for this has been conducted at The Albion Mount Medical Practice in Dewsbury.

Recently, Farah has also been involved in working with the University of Bradford to help mark the Pharmacy OSCEs and aims to continue working with students to help support and improve the future of pharmacy.

In her down time, Farah enjoys attending the gym, particularly lifting weights under the guidance of her personal trainer.

Abbreviations

ACBS	Advisory Committee on Borderline Substances
ACE	angiotensin-converting enzyme
ACEI	angiotensin-converting enzyme inhibitor
ACS	acute coronary syndrome
AF	atrial fibrillation
ALT DIE	alternate days
AV	arteriovenous
BD	twice daily
BMI	body mass index
BNF	*British National Formulary*
BNFC	*British National Formulary for Children*
BP	blood pressure
BPSA	British Pharmaceutical Students' Association
BSA	body surface area
BTS	British Thoracic Society
CCF	congestive/chronic cardiac failure
CD	controlled drug
CDC	US Centers for Disease Control and Prevention
CE	*conformité européenne*
CFC	chlorofluorocarbon
CHM	Commission on Human Medicines
CHMP	Committee for Medicinal Products for Human Use
CI	confidence interval or cumulative incidence
CKS	Clinical Knowledge Summaries
COX	cyclooxygenase
COPD	chronic obstructive pulmonary disease
CPD	continuing professional development
CPPE	Centre for Pharmacy Postgraduate Education
CrCl	creatinine clearance (mL/min)
CSM	Committee on Safety of Medicines
CYT	cytochrome
DigCl	digoxin clearance (L/h)
DMARD	disease-modifying antirheumatic drug
DNG	discount not given
DPF	*Dental Practitioners' Formulary*
DPI	dry-powder inhaler
EC	enteric-coated
ECG	electrocardiogram
EEA	European Economic Area
eGFR	estimated glomerular filtration rate
EHC	emergency hormonal contraception

F1	Foundation Year 1
FEV1	forced expiratory volume in 1 second
GP	general practitioner
GP6D	glucose-6-phosphate dehydrogenase
GPhC	General Pharmaceutical Council
GSL	general sales list
GTN	glyceryl trinitrate
HbA1c	glycated haemoglobin
HDU	high dependency unit
HIV	human immunodeficiency virus
HR	heart rate
HRT	hormone replacement therapy
IBS	irritable bowel syndrome
IBW	ideal body weight
IDA	industrial denatured alcohol
IM	intramuscular
INR	international normalised ratio
IV	intravenous
IUD	intrauterine device
MAOI	monoamine oxidase inhibitor
MD	maximum single dose
MDD	maximum daily dose
MDI	metered-dose inhaler
MDU	to be used as directed
MEP	*Medicines, Ethics and Practice guide*
MHRA	Medicines and Healthcare products Regulatory Agency
MMR	measles, mumps and rubella
M/R	modified-release
MRSA	methicillin-resistant *Staphylococcus aureus*
MUPS	multiple-unit pellet system
MUR	Medicines Use Review
NHS	National Health Service
NICE	National Institute for Health and Care Excellence
NMS	New Medicines Service
NRLS	National Reporting and Learning System
NSAIDs	non-steroidal anti-inflammatory drugs
OC	oral contraceptive
OD	*omni die* (every day)
OM	*omni mane* (every morning)
ON	*omni nocte* (every night)
OP	original pack
OPAT	outpatient parenteral antibacterial therapy
ORT	oral rehydration therapy

OTC	over-the-counter
P	pharmacy
PAGB	Proprietary Association of Great Britain
PCT	primary care trust
PHE	Public Health England
PIL	patient information leaflet
pMDI	pressurised metered-dose inhaler
PMR	patient medical record
POM	prescription-only medicine
POM-V	prescription-only medicine – veterinarian
POM-VPS	prescription-only medicine – veterinarian, pharmacist, suitably qualified person
PPIs	proton pump inhibitors
PRN	when required
PSA	prostate-specific antigen
PSNC	Pharmaceutical Services Negotiating Committee
QDS	*quarter die sumendum* (to be taken four times daily)
RCT	randomised controlled trial
RE	right eye
RPS	Royal Pharmaceutical Society (formerly RPSGB)
SARSS	Suspected Adverse Reaction Surveillance Scheme
SCRIPT	Standard Computerised Revalidation Instrument for Prescribing and Therapeutics
SeCr	serum creatinine
SGLT2	sodium (Na+)/glucose co-transporter 2
SHO	senior house officer
SIGN	Scottish Intercollegiate Guidelines Network
SLS	selected list scheme
SOP	standard operating procedure
SPC	summary of product characteristics
SSRI	selective serotonin reuptake inhibitor
ST	an isoelectric line after the QRS complex of an ECG
STAT	immediately
TCA	tricyclic antidepressant
TDS	three times a day
TIA	transient ischaemic attack
TPN	total parenteral nutrition
TSDA	trade-specific denatured alcohol
U&E	urea and electrolyte count
UTI	urinary tract infection
VITAL	Virtual Interactive Teaching And Learning
WHO	World Health Organization

High Weighted Questions

☐ **A** Amlodipine
☐ **B** Doxazosin
☐ **C** Indapamide
☐ **D** losartan
☐ **E** Ramipril
☐ **F** Spironolactone

For questions 1 – 5:

For the questions below, select the most likely medication. Each option may be used once, more than once or not at all.

1   You are a prescribing pharmacist working in General Practice. Mrs CM, an African Caribbean woman (52 years), visits your practice. She came in a week ago complaining of dizziness and headaches. The GP carried out a full clinical assessment and his only concern was her blood pressure. At the start of the consultation, it was 165/92 and towards the end of the consultation it was 159/80. The GP provided lifestyle advice and requested she monitors her blood pressure at home twice a day for a week and provide the readings. She returns today with the readings, and you calculate an average at 158/96. She has no other co-morbidities. Lifestyle advice has been reiterated to the patient. What is the most appropriate drug for this patient?

2   Mr JL, a Caucasian man (54 years), comes into your pharmacy. He is requesting a cough mixture for a dry cough that he has had for over two weeks. He informs you that he has started a blood pressure medication a few weeks ago too and isn't sure whether it is related. He informs you that he takes nil other prescribed medication. Which hypertensive medication from the list is most likely to cause a dry cough?

3   Mr JL is referred to his GP regarding his dry cough. The GP stops his current medication. Which hypertensive medication from the list is the most appropriate for the GP to switch to?

4   You are a prescribing pharmacist in General Practice. Mr WS, a Caucasian man (66 years), with a history of diabetes and hypertension comes into your practice for a routine blood pressure check and routine blood tests. He is currently taking anti-hypertensive medication and complains of swelling in his ankles. What is the most likely medication to cause this symptom?

5   Mrs EP, an Asian woman (58 years) with a BMI of 40, has come into your hypertension clinic. She is currently taking:
    • Amlodipine 5mg tablets – Take ONE daily
    • Metformin 500mg tablets – Take ONE twice a day
    • Paracetamol 500mg tablets – Take ONE or TWO up to four times a day WHEN REQUIRED
    • Ramipril 10mg Capsules – Take ONE daily

    You check her blood pressure, it is 160/92. You discuss her lifestyle and offer lifestyle advice. You proceed to check her blood pressure again and it is 159/94. At this stage, what is the most appropriate anti-hypertensive to add?

6   Mrs EP returns a few weeks later for a follow up in your hypertension clinic. She states she is well in herself since starting the new medication. You check her blood pressure, it is 149/90. You discuss lifestyle advice again and take another BP reading, it is 148/89. You seek advice from the GP, and she advises to consider the initiation of spironolactone. What do you need to ensure before prescribing spironolactone?

    ☐ A Calcium is ≤2.5
    ☐ B Creatinine is ≤84
    ☐ C Potassium is ≤4.5
    ☐ D Sodium is ≤137
    ☐ E Urea is ≤ 6.7

7   Miss LM (29 years) is a Caucasian woman and is currently having manic episodes associated with her bipolar disorder. The neurologist decides to commence the patient on sodium valproate 1g in the morning and 1.5g in the evening. The neurologist has requested that the pharmacists speak to the patient with regards to risks as he did not have time during his consultation. Which of the following statements is FALSE?

- [ ] **A** If sodium valproate is taken during pregnancy, up to 4 in 10 babies are at risk of developmental disorders, and approximately 1 in 10 are at risk of birth defects
- [ ] **B** Patient is of a childbearing age and therefore sodium valproate should not be prescribed unless there is no suitable alterative treatment
- [ ] **C** Sodium valproate 1g in the morning and 1.5g in the evening is not the appropriate dose in prescribing for mania associated with bipolar disorder
- [ ] **D** The GP can prescribe the sodium valproate providing the GP discusses pregnancy risks and ensures if the patient is sexually active, that contraception is in place to prevent pregnancy
- [ ] **E** The use of sodium valproate in pregnancy is contraindicated for bipolar disorder and must only be considered for epilepsy if there is no suitable alternative treatment

8   Mr AR, a 45-year-old Asian man, has a history of hypertension and is struggling to sleep at night following the passing of his wife. He has come to your community pharmacy with a prescription for zopiclone 7.5mg tablets – Take ONE at bedtime (56 tablets). What do you need to alert the GP to before issuing the prescription?

- [ ] **A** Advise GP that prescribing zopiclone is inappropriate for this patient given his age
- [ ] **B** Advise GP that zopiclone is contraindicated in this patient
- [ ] **C** Advise GP that zopiclone is only for short-term use for up to 4 weeks
- [ ] **D** Advise GP to commence patient on a reduced dose of zopiclone, 3.75mg for up to 4 weeks and uptitrate if necessary to 7.5mg based on the patients response
- [ ] **E** Advise GP to prescribe an oral solution because it is more cost effective

9   Ms AH, a 66-year-old Caucasian woman, presents to your community pharmacy. She has been diagnosed with gastro-oesophageal reflux disease and depression, and presents with a prescription as follows:
- Lansoprazole 15mg capsules – Take ONE daily (28)
- Escitalopram 20mg tablets – Take ONE daily (28)

Which statement is TRUE regarding this prescription?

☐ **A** Escitalopram 20mg tablets should be switched to citalopram 20mg tablets as it is more cost effective

☐ **B** Escitalopram and lansoprazole interact when taken together, there is an increased risk of bleeds

☐ **C** Escitalopram is contraindicated in patients with gastro-oesophageal reflux disease

☐ **D** Lansoprazole 15mg is a low dose, the doctor should consider lansoprazole 30mg to provide effective gastro protection

☐ **E** The dose of escitalopram should be reduced to 10mg daily in patients older than 65

10 Miss LW, a 29-year-old Caucasian woman, has been initiated on lithium therapy for bipolar affective disorder. She had her bloods taken 12 hours after her dose. You check her bloods to ensure her result was in the narrow therapeutic range. What is the narrow therapeutic range for this patient?

☐ **A** 0.2 – 1mmol/L
☐ **B** 0.4 – 1mmol/L
☐ **C** 0.6 – 1mmol/L
☐ **D** 0.7 – 1mmol/L
☐ **E** 0.8 – 1mmol/L

11 Mrs TA, a 51-year-old Caucasian woman, presents to the community pharmacy for the first time. She presents with a fever, sore throat and is complaining of mouth ulcers. She took a Covid PCR test, and the results returned as negative. She is wondering whether you could suggest some good remedies to help with her symptoms. She shows you her current list of medications as she has not been to your pharmacy before, and she is currently taking:

- Fluoxetine 20mg capsules – ONE daily (28)
- Carbamazepine 100mg tablets – ONE twice a day (56)
- Cimetidine 400mg – ONE twice a day for four weeks then reduce to ONE daily (56)

What is the MOST appropriate course of management for this patient?

☐ **A** Advise the patient to increase their fluid intake and rest. Suggest paracetamol for the fever, benzydamine throat spray for the sore throat and Bonjela for the mouth ulcers. If symptoms persist or worsen, the patient should consider visiting her GP.

☐ B Advise the patient to attend A&E as she may need a blood test.

☐ C Advise the patient to see her GP immediately – it is likely that the medication she is taking is causing her symptoms.

☐ D Advise the patient to take ibuprofen 400mg three times a day after food as it will help to reduce the inflammation causing the sore throat and help to regulate the body temperature.

☐ E Refer the patient to the walk-in-centre for a full clinical assessment. The patient may have exudate on her tonsils which could be contributing to her sore throat and overall illness.

12   Mr BW, a 64-year-old Caucasian man, comes into your community pharmacy complaining of dizziness, confusion, and dry mouth. He mentions that he hasn't been able to pass stools for three days and is struggling to urinate. He informs you that the GP recently started him on a new medication, and he wonders whether that could be the cause of him feeling this way. Which drug is most likely to contribute to these symptoms?

☐ A Amitriptyline

☐ B Carvediol

☐ C Clonidine

☐ D Digoxin

☐ E Lansoprazole

13   Mrs SS, a 45-year-old Asian woman, comes into your community pharmacy with a prescription for:

• Codeine 30mg tablets – Take ONE or TWO four times a day when required (200)

You notice that she takes this medication regularly. Which statement is FALSE regarding this patient's medication?

☐ A Codeine can cause drowsiness and may affect performance of skilled tasks, e.g. driving.

☐ B Codeine is contraindicated in breast feeding mothers.

☐ C Codeine is contraindicated in patients of any age who are known to be ultra-rapid metabolisers of codeine (CYP2D6 ultra-rapid metabolisers).

☐ D Codeine is suitable in children (under 18) who undergo the removal of tonsils or adenoids for the treatment of obstructive sleep apnoea.

☐ E Prolonged use of opioid analgesics may lead to drug dependence and addiction, even at therapeutic doses.

For questions 14 – 18, select the most likely medication. Each option may be used once, more than once or not at all.

☐ A Empagliflozin
☐ B Gliclazide
☐ C Hetformin
☐ D Pioglitazone
☐ E Sitagliptin

14 Mrs KA, a 66-year-old Caucasian woman, has just been counselled on how to recognise the signs and symptoms of diabetic ketoacidosis after being prescribed a drug from the list. Which of the drugs is this most likely to be?

15 Miss OH, a 25-year-old Asian woman, comes into your pharmacy with a prescription which she says she needs to take for her 'polycystic ovary syndrome.' Which medication is most likely being prescribed here?

16 Mr HO, a 69-year-old Caucasian man, presents in A&E with hypoglycaemia. He is diabetic and is in CKD3. Which medication carries the greatest risk of causing the hypoglycaemic incident?

17 Mr PC, a 55-year-old Asian man, presents to A&E with severe abdominal pain, nausea, and vomiting. The doctors diagnose this patient with pancreatitis. Which of the medication is most likely to have caused the symptoms?

18 Which of the antidiabetic drugs listed increases the risk of heart failure when given with insulin?

19 Mrs HA, a 52-year-old Caucasian woman, has been receiving prednisolone 60mg daily for a week for 'giant cell arteiritis with visual disturbances'. The patient informs the doctor that her vision seems to have restored and

she is beginning to feel a lot better. The doctor wants to begin reducing the dose of prednisolone. Which statement below is FALSE in relation to prednisolone withdrawal?

☐ A Abrupt withdrawal after a prolonged period can lead to acute adrenal insufficiency, hypotension, or death.

☐ B Abrupt withdrawal after a weeks' worth of prednisolone can lead to hypovolaemic shock.

☐ C Abrupt withdrawal can be associated with fever, myalgia, arthralgia, rhinitis, conjunctivitis, painful itchy skin nodules and weight loss.

☐ D Mrs HA should have her prednisolone reduced gradually to a maintenance dose of 7.5 – 10mg daily. She would require this dose for at least two years.

☐ E The magnitude and speed of dose reduction in corticosteroid withdrawal should be determined on a case-by-case basis, taking into consideration the underlying condition that is being treated, and individual patient factors such as the likelihood of relapse and the duration of corticosteroid treatment.

20 A child is brought into your pharmacy by his mother. She shows you that her son has red sores with orange crusts around his mouth which she is concerned about. On examination, what is the most likely presentation?

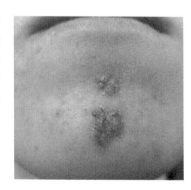

Reproduced from James Heilman, MD under the following CC BY-SA 4.0 license, https://creativecommons.org/licenses/by-sa/4.0/deed.en.

☐ A Chickenpox
☐ B Herpes simplex
☐ C Impetigo
☐ D Slapped cheek syndrome
☐ E Tinea corporis

21 You are a hospital pharmacist and the pharmacy team have requested that you complete an audit on the use of broad-spectrum antibiotics being

used for antimicrobial stewardship. Which listed below is NOT a broad-spectrum antibiotic?

☐ A Cefalexin
☐ B Ciprofloxacin
☐ C Co-amoxiclav
☐ D Levofloxacin
☐ E Vancomycin

22 Miss FN, a 21-year-old Caucasian woman, presents with a painful, inflamed red lump on the skin with a visible red line spreading out of it. She explains she has been gardening and felt something bite her. On examination, the doctor confirms it is an infectious bite. She tells you that she is allergic to penicillin as it gives her a rash. What is the most appropriate antibiotic to prescribe for this patient?

☐ A Co-amoxiclav
☐ B Doxycycline
☐ C Flucloxacillin
☐ D Nitrofurantoin
☐ E Trimethoprim

23 Miss BH, a 31-year-old Asian woman who has a penicillin allergy, has been given a prescription for:
• Lansoprazole 30mg – ONE twice a day (14)
• Clarithromycin 500mg – ONE twice a day (14)
• Metronidazole 400mg – ONE twice a day (14)
What is she likely being treated for?

☐ A *Arcanobacterium haemolyticum*
☐ B *Clostridium difficile*
☐ C *Helicobacter pylori*
☐ D *Legionella pneumophilia*
☐ E *Nesseria meningitidis*

24 Mr AR, a 20-year-old Afro-Caribbean male, presents to your community pharmacy with a red, watery eye (left eye). He advises that it is worse in the morning as it is sticky and filled with 'yellow gunk' which he cleans

with cool boiled water and a clean flannel, as per advice from his mother. He has had these symptoms for two days and it seems to be getting worse. You conclude that this is potentially bacterial conjunctivitis. Which statement is FALSE with regards to treatment options in conjunctivitis?

☐ A 1st line treatment is chloramphenicol 0.5% eye drops – 1 drop 2 hourly for 2 days, reducing to 4 hourly as the infection improves for 7 days.

☐ B 2nd line treatment is fusidic acid 1% eye drops twice a day, continue for 48 hours after resolution.

☐ C Fusidic acid has a significant price increase compared to chloramphenicol and should only be used when absolutely necessary, when chloramphenicol is not suitable.

☐ D Swab all people who are sexually active for gonococcal and chlamydial infection who have conjunctivitis that persists for 14 days despite treatment.

☐ E Swab the eye for culture and sensitivity if infective conjunctivitis is not resolving after 7 days.

25 Some patients who are at risk of exacerbations of chronic obstructive pulmonary disease may have antibiotics to keep at home as part of their exacerbation action plan. Which of the following statements is TRUE about rescue packs?

☐ A All exacerbations are caused by bacteria and this is the reason patients with COPD are supplied rescue packs.

☐ B If a patient has a penicillin allergy then an appropriate rescue pack medication would be co-amoxiclav 500/125 three times a day for 5 days + prednisolone 30mg once daily for 5 days.

☐ C If the patient is taking frequent rescue packs they should be reviewed with the GP. The GP should review prescribing of rescue packs, review antibiotic choice including sputum cultures and sensitivities and consider if symptoms are masking anything more sinister like lung cancer.

☐ D If there are more than 2 issues in the last 12 months then the patient needs to see a GP.

☐ E Rescue packs can only be given if a sputum sample suggests that the patient has an infection.

26 Miss UI, a 52-year-old Caucasian woman, presents to the out of hours
walk-in-centre complaining of pain and burning when she is urinating.
She explains it feels like there is a pulling sensation and despite her
need to go to the toilet, when she does go there is very little voiding.
The advanced nurse practitioner (ANP) carries out a urine dipstick and
finds neutrophils, leucocytes, and traces of blood (positive). The patient
advises that she is allergic to penicillin, and that she has been told by
the GP she has chronic kidney disease stage 3. The ANP asks for your
advice so you check her clinical records and find that her recent eGFR
is 48ml/min. What is the most appropriate medication to describe for
this patient?

☐ A Cefalexin
☐ B Co-amoxiclav
☐ C Fosfomycin
☐ D Nitrofurantoin
☐ E Pivmecillinam

The next four questions are based on the same list of options, but different
scenarios. Each option may be used once, more than once or not at all.

☐ A Alpha-blockers
☐ B Angiotensin converting enzyme inhibitor (ACEi)
☐ C Angiotensin receptor blockers (ARB)s
☐ D Beta-blockers
☐ E Calcium channel blockers
☐ F Loop diuretics
☐ G Potassium sparing diuretics/mineralocorticoid receptor antagonists
☐ H Thiazide-like diuretic

27 A 52-year-old woman was diagnosed with stage 1 hypertension six
months ago, with an average home blood pressure reading of 149/94
mmHg. She was thus prescribed ramipril as 1st line treatment as per the
NICE guidelines. The practice pharmacist has now received a discharge
letter for this patient which shows she suffered a delayed angioedema
reaction to this drug. Which other class of medication should also be
avoided for this patient?

28 A 66-year-old male patient with type 2 diabetes was prescribed lisinopril 5mg as a renoprotective agent. After 3 weeks, he contacts the diabetes nurse to discuss what he thinks may be a potential side effect of the lisinopril. He mentions that he has a dry, tickly cough which does not seem to be settling with the cough mixture he bought from the pharmacy last week. Which class of medication would be a suitable alternative?

29 A 76-year-old woman was diagnosed with heart failure (HF) one year ago. She was started on ramipril and bisoprolol which were gradually titrated to a maximum tolerated dose of 5mg and 7.5mg respectively. She has a follow up appointment with the HF nurse and reports ongoing symptoms of fatigue, a chronic cough and breathlessness. Her most recent eGFR is 65ml/min and potassium levels are 3mmol/L. What is the most likely next class of medicines that the HF nurse will prescribe from?

30 A 60-year-old woman with diagnosed heart failure, books a GP appointment to discuss some symptoms she is experiencing. She developed severe pain in her big toe which started suddenly yesterday. The toe is also red, hot, and painful to touch. Her current list of medications is:
- Bisoprolol 1.25mg
- Furosemide 20mg
- Lisinopril 2.5mg
- Spironolactone 25mg

From which class of drugs is the medication that caused her new symptoms?

31 A 27-year-old female has been prescribed sertraline 50mg for generalised anxiety disorder (GAD) one week ago. She reports back to say it is not working and that she wishes to try an alternative. What is the most appropriate next step?

☐ A Advise her that it may take 2-3 weeks before she notices any improvement
☐ B Continue sertraline and add in propranolol 40mg TDS
☐ C Increase sertraline to 100mg OD
☐ D Refer for counselling
☐ E Stop sertraline and trial propranolol 40mg TDS

32 A 75-year-old male has been taking citalopram 30mg OD for one year. He visits his GP to discuss a change in his circumstances which have meant that the citalopram is now not controlling his depression. The GP decides to gradually increase his citalopram to 40mg and to review in 2 weeks. His current list of medications is:

- Aspirin 75mg OD
- Lansoprazole 15mg OD
- Citalopram 40mg OD
- Amlodipine 5mg OD
- Simvastatin 20mg ON

Which one of the following is a correct statement regarding this treatment?

☐ A Citalopram above the dose of 20mg in the elderly is not appropriate
☐ B Citalopram should be switched to fluoxetine
☐ C Lansoprazole strength should be higher for gastroprotection
☐ D The combination of medication and doses are safe to prescribe
☐ E There is an interaction between aspirin and citalopram, therefore aspirin needs to stop

33 A 35-year-old woman has been diagnosed with epilepsy and is prescribed carbamazepine for her focal tonic-clonic seizures by her neurologist. She then books a telephone appointment with the GP regarding starting a suitable contraceptive tablet, who in turn seeks your advice. Which one of the following is a suitable form of contraception?

☐ A Cerazette tablets (desogestrel 75mcg)
☐ B Desogestrel 75mg OD
☐ C Evra patches (ethinylestradiol 33.9mcg, norelgestromin 203mcg)
☐ D Levonorgestrel intrauterine system
☐ E Microgynon tablets (ethinylestradiol 30mcg with levonorgestrel 150mcg)

34 A 56-year-old Muslim man with type 2 diabetes, has recently been switched over from oral anti-diabetic drugs to lantus 100units/ml solution for injection prefilled SoloStar pens. He has an appointment with the diabetes nurse to discuss how he will manage his insulin during the

month of Ramadhan. His current dose is 15units BD. What is the most appropriate advice to give this patient?

☐ A Increase the units for both doses as fasting can cause an increase in your blood glucose
☐ B Revert back to oral anti-diabetics
☐ C Skip both doses of insulin as he will be fasting anyway
☐ D Take the morning dose and reduce the evening dose by 50%
☐ E Take the morning dose only

35 Mrs AF is a 46-year-old woman who attends for a routine review with her GP. She mentions that she has symptoms including weight gain, although her appetite has decreased. She has also been feeling exceptionally tired over the last year and struggling to keep warm despite having the heating on at home on most days. The GP notices that her full blood count (FBC) was actioned recently and the results for this had come back normal so suspects a potential diagnosis of an underlying endocrinology condition. What should the GP expect to see in her blood test results?

☐ A Low ferritin levels
☐ B Low folate levels
☐ C Raised HbA1c levels
☐ D Raised TSH and low T4
☐ E Raised TSH and T4 normal

36 A 25-year-old international student who is temporarily registered at the GP surgery, is prescribed colecalciferol 50,000-unit capsules once a week for 6 weeks as her blood test showed a deficiency in vitamin D. She has misunderstood the dosage instructions and ended up taking one capsule a day instead. You were able to note this because she has called the community pharmacy requesting a further prescription and has 'ran out of medication.' Which one of the following is an appropriate test to monitor due to the above situation?

☐ A eGFR
☐ B Liver function tests
☐ C Serum calcium levels
☐ D Serum sodium levels
☐ E Thyroid stimulating hormone levels

37 A 44-year-old woman (Mrs BL) with excessive polydipsia and polyuria has been diagnosed with diabetes insipidus. She has been prescribed treatment by her endocrinologist. With this medication, if she is underdosed she will develop polyuria and thirst, if overdosed it will cause confusion due to hyponatraemia. Which one of the following medications has this patient been prescribed?

☐ **A** Bendroflumethiazide tablets
☐ **B** Canagliflozin tablets
☐ **C** Desmopressin nasal spray
☐ **D** Ibuprofen gel
☐ **E** Metformin tablets

38 Mrs FS (33 years) comes into the community pharmacy to seek advice regarding malaria prevention and sunscreens. You are the responsible pharmacist. She informs you that she will be travelling with her family (her husband and three children). They will be taking a trip to Nigeria over the summer to visit family. Along with providing a prescription for anti-malarial tablets, the GP has also advised her to ensure she uses insect repellent which contains >20% DEET concentrations. Which one of the following is true regarding DEET and sunscreen application?

☐ **A** Apply sunscreen SPF 15-30 and then DEET at >20% concentration
☐ **B** Apply the DEET at 20% concentration first and then use the sunscreen 30-50 SPF
☐ **C** DEET dilutes sunscreen so apply SPF 30-50 first, then DEET at >20% concentration
☐ **D** DEET dilutes sunscreen so avoid using it, as the anti-malarial tablets should be enough
☐ **E** DEET does not affect sunscreen, so it does not matter which way round it is used

39 A 38-year-old woman comes into the pharmacy to seek advice about some symptoms she has been experiencing. She mentions that she has had a burning sensation on the left side of her back and generally feeling a bit unwell. Three days later a rash has come up on the area that was burning, which her husband has noticed and recommended she get advice for. He asks that you take a look in the consultation room, and this is what you see:

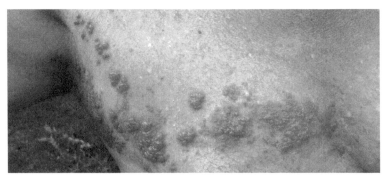

What is the most likely diagnosis?

- ☐ A Candidal infection
- ☐ B Chickenpox
- ☐ C Contact dermatitis
- ☐ D Herpes simplex virus (HSV) infection
- ☐ E Shingles

40 A 55-year-old male patient has had a total splenectomy and due to the ongoing high risk of pneumococcal infection, is recommended prophylactic antibiotics lifelong. He previously trialled penicillin V, came up in a rash and had a tingling sensation in the throat. Which one of the following would be the most appropriate prophylactic antibiotics?

- ☐ A Amoxicillin 500mg BD
- ☐ B Azithromycin 250MG Monday, Wednesday and Friday
- ☐ C Erythromycin 500mg BD
- ☐ D Lymecycline 408mg OD
- ☐ E Phenoxymethylpenicillin 250mg BD

41 A 67-year-old woman has handed in a urine sample to her routine nurse to check as part of her annual diabetes and chronic kidney disease (CKD) review. She has known stage 4 CKD. She mentions increased frequency and urgency of urination, burning and also cloudy urine. The sample has tested positive for nitrites and leucocytes. She has no allergies. Which of the following antibiotics should be prescribed as first-line for this patient?

☐ A Flucloxacillin 500mg QDS for 3 days
☐ B Nitrofurantoin 100mg BD for 7 days
☐ C Nitrofurantoin MR 100mg BD 3 days
☐ D Trimethoprim 100mg OD for 3 days
☐ E Trimethoprim 200mg BD for 3 days

42 You are working as a hospital pharmacist and have been asked by a clinician for advice on managing a side effect of a medication. A patient began experiencing nightmares a week after starting a beta-blocker. Which of the following beta-blockers has the patient most likely been initiated on?

☐ A Atenolol
☐ B Celiprolol
☐ C Nadolol
☐ D Propranolol
☐ E Sotalol

43 A 60-year-old woman has been newly diagnosed with severe aortic stenosis following a doppler echo examination. She has a past medical history of atrial fibrillation, hypertension and QRISK score of 20%. The patient had a non-ST elevated myocardial infarction 9 months ago. You note the following results in the patient's medical record:
• Blood pressure: 130/88mmHg | heart rate: 70 bpm
• CHA2DS2-VASc score: 3
• eGFR: 85mL/min/1.73m2
• ORBIT score: 1
• Serum creatinine: 90 micromol/L
• Weight: 80kg

Which of the following repeat medications would be unsuitable to continue following the new diagnosis?

☐ A Amlodipine
☐ B Apixaban
☐ C Atorvastatin
☐ D Bisoprolol
☐ E Ramipril

44 A 68-year-old man with a medical history of hypertension has been admitted to hospital after having slurred speech, weakness of the left arm and a severe headache. 12 hours after the onset, the symptoms have resolved, and the patient was subsequently diagnosed with transient ischaemic attack (TIA). The patient has previously not been able to tolerate clopidogrel. Which of the following would be the most appropriate for the secondary prevention of a TIA?

☐ A Aspirin 300mg tablets
☐ B Aspirin 75mg tablets
☐ C Clopidogrel 75mg tablets
☐ D Dipyridamole 200mg modified-release capsules
☐ E Dipyridamole 200mg modified-release capsules plus aspirin 75mg tablets

45 A 28-years-old male patient has been inhaling nitrous oxide recreationally. He started inhaling the gas 3 years ago after a night out with some friends. After experiencing pain and tingling in the toes and fingers he has decided to stop. He acknowledges the harm of nitrous oxide and would like to reduce the number of cannisters he uses before stopping altogether. Which of the following stage of the Prochaska & DiClemente cycle of change is the patient currently at?

☐ A Action
☐ B Contemplation
☐ C Maintenance
☐ D Pre-contemplation
☐ E Preparation

46 You are a practice pharmacist reviewing acute medication requests. A 26-year-old female is 18 weeks pregnant and is requesting a particular anti-emetic. Upon reviewing the medication requested, you notice a medication alert recommending the use of the medication for a maximum of five days and to avoid in the first trimester due to a small risk of congenital abnormalities. Which of the following medication has the patient likely requested?

☐ A Cyclizine
☐ B Domperidone

☐ C Metoclopramide
☐ D Ondansetron
☐ E Promethazine

47 A 45-year-old female is due to undergo a total abdominal hysterectomy next week. Undergoing a major surgery like this may require temporarily stopping medication. Which of the following medication should be stopped 24 hours before the surgery?

☐ A Amisulpride
☐ B Haloperidol
☐ C Lithium
☐ D Methadone
☐ E Rotigotine

48 A 19-year-old male has been diagnosed with type 1 diabetes following a urine ketone and blood glucose test in hospital. A specialist diabetic nurse has instructed the patient on how to use his insulin but failed to mention the blood glucose targets to aim for. You are the ward pharmacist and have been asked to clarify the blood glucose targets. What is the optimum blood glucose target level on waking in patients with type 1 diabetes?

☐ A 4–7mmol/L
☐ B 4–9mmol/L
☐ C 5–7mmol/L
☐ D 5–9mmol/L
☐ E 7–11mmol/L

49 A 48-year-old male patient has been referred to your community pharmacy for a Community Pharmacist Consultation Service (CPCS). He presents with 3-4 small, round mouth ulcers. The patient would like to try medication to relieve the discomfort. You note the patients is taking the following medications:

- Atorvastatin 20mg once daily
- Carbimazole 10mg once daily
- Colecalciferol 800 units daily
- Levothyroxine 75 microgram daily

Which of the following would be the most appropriate course of action?

☐ A Do not treat over-the-counter; see GP if unresolved within 7 days
☐ B Refer to accident & emergency (A&E)
☐ C Refer to GP urgently
☐ D Treat with over-the-counter medicine and provide advice prognosis
☐ E Treat with over-the-counter medicine; see GP if unresolved within 7 days

50 A 40-year-old male patient has been identified to have uncontrolled type 2 diabetes following a diabetic review. You are the practice pharmacist and have been asked to recommend a suitable antidiabetic medicine for dual-therapy. You note the patient has a history of bladder cancer, stable heart failure and was recently treated for Fournier's gangrene. He also has a phobia of needles. The patient's latest BMI was recorded at $31kg/m^2$ and recent HbA1C was 73mmol/L. He is currently taking the following medications:

- Atorvastatin 20mg once a day
- Metformin 1g twice a day
- Ramipril 2.5mg once a day

Which of the medication would be the most appropriate to recommend?

☐ A Canagliflozin
☐ B Exenatide
☐ C Glimepiride
☐ D Linagliptin
☐ E Pioglitazone

51 You are a prescribing pharmacist operating a minor ailments clinic. A 26-year-old female patient presents with urinary urgency and a burning sensation upon passing urine. A urine dipstick test is positive for nitrites and reveals moderate amounts of leukocytes in the urine. Based on your clinical assessment you diagnose the patient with a lower urinary tract infection. She is currently 10 weeks pregnant and has a mild penicillin allergy (rash); she takes no regular medication. Her eGFR has been recorded at >90ml/min. Which of the following would be the most appropriate antibiotic for this patient?

☐ A Amoxicillin 500mg TDS for 7 days
☐ B Cefalexin 500mg BD for 7 days
☐ C Nitrofurantoin MR 100mg BD for 3 days
☐ D Pivmecillinam 400mg for 1 dose, then 200mg 8 hourly to a total of 10 tablets
☐ E Trimethoprim 200mg BD for 3 days

52 An 83-year-old male has been referred to hospital by his GP due to presenting with cholestatic jaundice. In the medication history, it was noted the patient had completed a 14-day course of antibiotics a month ago. You are the ward pharmacist reviewing the patient and you suspect the recent antibiotic may be the cause of the patient's symptoms. Which of the following antibiotic is likely to be responsible for this adverse effect?

☐ A Amoxicillin
☐ B Ciprofloxacin
☐ C Doxycycline
☐ D Flucloxacillin
☐ E Gentamicin

53 A mother has brought her 4-year-old daughter to A&E with a suspected case of meningitis. The child has a rash with tiny purple spots that are firm when pressure has been applied. She is lethargic and has a temperature of 39°C. It is noted the child has previously had an immediate anaphylactic reaction to penicillin and cephalosporins. You are the on-call hospital pharmacist and have been asked to recommend an appropriate antibiotic for this patient. Which of the following antibiotics would be the most appropriate to recommend for this patient?

☐ A Benzylpenicillin IV
☐ B Cefotaxime IV
☐ C Chloramphenicol IV
☐ D Teicoplanin oral
☐ E Tigecycline IV

Questions 54-58 will consider relevant therapeutic drug parameters. Which statement is the most APPROPRIATE for the following drugs?

☐ **A** Apixaban
☐ **B** Aspirin
☐ **C** Clopidogrel
☐ **D** Dipyridamole
☐ **E** Warfarin

54 Requires dosage adjustment if creatinine clearance falls below 29ml/min?

55 Is indicated for stroke prophylaxis in patients with prosthetic heart valves?

56 Concomitant prescription of omeprazole should be avoided?

57 Is most likely to cause hypotension?

58 Can be crushed and mixed with apple juice?

59 Mr ID, a 43-year-old white male, has recently been diagnosed with hypertension following home blood pressure monitoring readings of 146/92mmHg. He has seen the practice nurse and been given lifestyle advice. He is booked onto your hypertension clinic to discuss initial treatment options. He has no other medical history of note. Which is the most APPROPRIATE drug of choice?

☐ **A** ACE inhibitor
☐ **B** Beta-blocker
☐ **C** Calcium channel blocker
☐ **D** Loop diuretic
☐ **E** Thiazide-like diuretic

60 Mr ID returns to your clinic 2 weeks later for a review. What monitoring is required at this review?

☐ **A** Blood pressure and serum magnesium
☐ **B** Blood pressure, heart rate and liver function
☐ **C** Blood pressure, liver function and renal function
☐ **D** Blood pressure, renal function and electrolytes
☐ **E** Blood pressure, renal function and serum potassium

61 Mr OH, a 37-year-old man, visits your community pharmacy and asks for your advice on the back pain he has been experiencing. You do not recognise him and on checking your PMR, he is not a regular patient at your pharmacy. He explains he is a labourer and has been experiencing lower back pain for 3 months following a work-related injury. He has tried taking paracetamol PRN but this has not been effective. In what circumstances should you AVOID using an NSAID?

☐ A Concomitant drug therapy with another NSAID
☐ B Concomitant drug therapy with SSRI
☐ C Hypertension controlled to below 135/85mmHg with ramipril 10mg daily
☐ D Mild heart failure
☐ E Moderate renal impairment

62 Mr OH then tells you he is 'allergic' to ibuprofen; it gave him terrible heartburn. How do you proceed?

☐ A Advise him to take ibuprofen after food
☐ B Refer him to A and E
☐ C Refer him to his GP for further investigation
☐ D Refer him to his GP with a note suggesting prescribing naproxen
☐ E Refer him to his GP with a note suggesting prescribing naproxen plus lansoprazole 15mg daily

63 Dr FC would like your help in converting her patient currently taking co-codamol 30/500mg 2 tablets qds and buprenorphine 20mcg patch changed once weekly, with oramorph 10mg/5ml solution for breakthrough cancer pain. She estimates that she is currently taking 2.5ml qds but is still experiencing pain. Which of the following would you suggest Dr FC switches her patient to? You have access to the BNF - https://bnf.nice.org. uk/guidance/prescribing-in-palliative-care.html

☐ A Fentanyl '50' patch once weekly
☐ B Intravenous morphine 10mg tds
☐ C Intravenous morphine 20mg bd
☐ D Oral morphine M/R tablets 40mg bd
☐ E Oral morphine M/R tablets 50mg bd

64 Miss JN, a 24-year-old female, comes into the community pharmacy asking for advice about headaches she has been experiencing. She describes intense pain on one side of her head that is pulsing in nature. She usually feels nauseated but is rarely sick. She has recently noticed that she can also experience pins and needles in her hands before the headache comes on. You suspect migraines in this patient. Which statement is true regarding migraines?

☐ A Migraines are more prevalent in men

☐ B Prophylaxis may be initiated in primary care for pregnant or breastfeeding adults

☐ C The licenced dose of oral zolmitriptan for a migraine is 5mg taken as soon as possible after the onset of a migraine, followed by 5mg after at least 2 hours if required.

☐ D Triggers may include dehydration, irregular meals, tiredness, and stress

☐ E Triptans may be safely taken with SSRIs and MAOIs

For questions 65-67, choose the most APPROPRIATE drug:

☐ A Aminophylline

☐ B Carbamazepine

☐ C Crifampicin

☐ D Sertraline

☐ E Sodium valproate

65 Which is an inducer of the CYP3A4 enzyme?

66 Which is an inhibitor of the CYP3A4 enzyme?

67 Which increase the risk of digoxin toxicity when given together?

68 Mrs IT, a 43-year-old type-2 diabetic, comes into the community pharmacy complaining of regular episodes of irritability, severe hunger, shaking hands, and feeling like her heart is racing. You identify that she is experiencing a possible hypoglycaemic attack. You check your PMR and note that she is taking metformin 1g bd, glimepiride 4mg od, linagliptin 5mg daily, atorvastatin 40mg daily, amitriptyline 20mg nocte. Which of the following statements is TRUE?

    □ A An improvement in clinical signs and symptoms may precede an improvement in blood glucose level

    □ B Awareness of hypoglycaemia signs and symptoms and how to manage these should be assessed and reinforced at annual reviews with patients

    □ C Blood glucose targets can be relaxed for patients with impaired awareness of hypoglycaemia

    □ D Hypoglycaemia is defined as a blood glucose level of 2.5mmol/L or lower

    □ E Metformin is commonly associated with hypoglycaemia

69 Mrs IT, a 43-year-old, has been referred to you in your diabetes clinic (within primary care) by the community pharmacist following a consultation which picked up that Mrs IT has been experiencing mild hypoglycaemic events. Her HbA1c is 47mmol/L. You agree that her glimepiride dose should be reduced. In conversation, Mrs IT mentions symptoms of peripheral neuropathy. Which of the following is CORRECT?

    □ A Amitriptyline is not used in the management of peripheral neuropathy

    □ B Monoamine oxidase inhibitors can be used in the treatment of peripheral neuropathy

    □ C Neuropathic pain can respond to opioids

    □ D Pregabalin is not used in the management of peripheral neuropathy

    □ E Topical plasters are not usually indicated

70 You are a prescribing pharmacist in primary care. Mrs FS (a 56-year-old) with known hypothyroidism attends your surgery clinic following her annual blood test. The results are as follows:

- TSH: 3mU/L (0.4 – 4.0mU/L)
- Free T4: 11mU/L (9 – 24pmol/L)
- Free T3: 4.6pmol/L (3.5 – 7.8pmol/L)

The current dose of levothyroxine is 25mcg daily. She is experiencing no symptoms of overt hypothyroidism. Which of the following statements is true?

    □ A Mrs FS's TFTs should be re-checked in 3 months

    □ B Mrs FS's thyroxine dose should be increased

☐ C Mrs FS's thyroxine dose should be reduced

☐ D You should ensure Mrs FS has an appointment for her next annual blood test and advise to return if she experiences signs or symptoms of hypothyroidism

☐ E You should initiate liothyronine therapy

For the next three questions, select the most appropriate answer:

☐ A Alogliptin
☐ B Canagliflozin
☐ C Glimepiride
☐ D Glucagon
☐ E Humalog
☐ F Metformin
☐ G Pioglitazone
☐ H Repaglinide

71 Which is an oral therapy commonly associated with weight gain?

72 Which should not be used in those who have uninvestigated macroscopic haematuria?

73 Which is only licensed as a single therapy or in combination with metformin?

For the next four questions (74-77), select the most appropriate first line drug options. Each option may be used once, more than one or not at all.

Theme: Antibiotics

☐ A Amoxicillin
☐ B Doxycycline
☐ C Flucloxacillin
☐ D Nitrofurantoin
☐ E Terbinafine
☐ F Trimethoprim
☐ G Vancomycin
☐ H None of the above

74 Lower UTI in pregnant woman?

75 Cellulitis?

76 Onychomycosis on 1 toenail?

77 Acute bronchitis, systemically well and no co-morbidities?

78 Mrs KW (a 51-year-old female) has recently tested positive for *Helicobacter pylori* infection. She is penicillin allergic (rash) and is also taking the following regular medication: aspirin 75mg daily, clopidogrel 75mg daily, atorvastatin 80mg daily, bisoprolol 2.5mg daily, lansoprazole 15mg daily, ramipril 10mg daily and GTN spray PRN. Which option is the MOST appropriate to treat the *H. pylori* infection?

☐ **A** Lansoprazole 30mg bd, amoxicillin 1g bd, clarithromycin 500mg bd
☐ **B** Lansoprazole 30mg bd, amoxicillin 1g bd, metronidazole 400mg bd
☐ **C** Lansoprazole 30mg bd, clarithromycin 500mg bd, metronidazole 400mg bd
☐ **D** Omeprazole 40mg bd, amoxicillin 1g bd, metronidazole 400mg bd
☐ **E** Omeprazole 40mg bd, clarithromycin 500mg bd, metronidazole 400mg bd

79 Which of the following is a correct statement regarding *H. pylori* eradication therapy?

☐ **A** *H. pylori* is also associated with acute and chronic gastritis but NOT gastric cancer
☐ **B** *H. pylori* is one of the least common causes of peptic ulcer disease
☐ **C** NSAIDs do not have an additive effect
☐ **D** Presence should be confirmed before starting eradication therapy
☐ **E** All of the above are correct

80 Mr OL, an 83-year-old male, attends your respiratory clinic within primary care. He has COPD and is currently experiencing increased breathlessness affecting his ability to undertake his usual daily activities. His sputum which is usually a white colour is now yellow-green and thicker than usual. You check his medical record and note that Mr OL has recently had a course of amoxicillin for an unrelated infection. He has NKDA. How do you proceed?

- ☐ A Amoxicillin 500mg three times daily for 5 days
- ☐ B Amoxicillin 500mg three times daily for 5 days plus prednisolone 30mg daily for 5 days
- ☐ C Doxycycline 200mg on day 1, then 100mg on days 2-5 (total 5 day course)
- ☐ D Prednisolone 30mg daily for 5 days
- ☐ E Request a sputum sample for culture and susceptibility testing

81 Mr EB (65-years-old) is admitted onto the cardiovascular ward due to a recent myocardial infarction. You are the hospital clinical pharmacist on duty and are asked to review medication on discharge. Which of the following is a likely regime on discharge?

- ☐ A Ramipril, amlodipine, aspirin, furosemide and atorvastatin
- ☐ B Ramipril, bisoprolol, aspirin, clopidogrel and atorvastatin
- ☐ C Ramipril, bisoprolol, warfarin, aspirin and simvastatin
- ☐ D Ramipril, spironolactone, clopidogrel and atorvastatin
- ☐ E Ramipiril, warfarin, amlodipine, simvastatin and furosemide

82 Master JK (age 6 years) presents to the community pharmacy with mum. He is complaining of shortness of breath and is unable to complete sentences. Mum informs you that she checked his peak flow and it is less than 50% best. She is requiring an emergency supply of salbutamol as he has completely run out. You have access to pulse oximetry and note his oxygen levels are 90%, resp rate is 35/minute and his heart rate is 135 bpm. Which of the following statement is CORRECT?

- ☐ A This is a sign of life-threatening asthma and patient needs referral to A&E
- ☐ B This is a sign of moderate acute asthma and patient needs referral to A&E
- ☐ C This is a sign of moderate acute asthma and patient needs referral to the GP
- ☐ D This is a sign of severe acute asthma and patient needs referral to A&E
- ☐ E This is a sign of severe acute asthma and patient needs referral to the GP

83 Mr GH (45-years-old) presents to the GP complaining of shortness of breath, cough and purulent sputum. He has a well-established history of asthma. He has had multiple asthma exacerbations in the past. He presents today and the observations are as follows: 2 days cough, yellow sputum, temp – 37.2, oxygen saturation – 99%, peak flow 90% predicted, heart rate 62 and respiratory rate 16 breaths/minute, able to complete sentences, looks well and alert. Which of the following is the MOST appropriate action to take?

☐ A Prescribe amoxicillin 500mg TDS PO and prednisolone 40md OD PO (5 day course)
☐ B Prescribe amoxicillin 500mg TDS PO and prednisolone 40md OD PO (7 day course)
☐ C Prescribe amoxicillin 500mg TDS PO for 5 days
☐ D Prescribe prednisolone 40md OD PO for 5 days
☐ E No prescription needed due to likely viral indication

84 Miss KC visits her practice nurse for an annual asthma review. Her current asthma medications are salbutamol easi-breath 100milligrams 1-2puffs inh PRN and Fostair 200/6micrograms 2 puffs BD. She advises the practice nurse that her asthma is still affecting her daily activities and that she is also sometimes waking at night with the symptoms. Which of the following is the appropriate plan of action?

☐ A Check inhaler technique and add montelukast 10mg OD
☐ B Check inhaler technique and add prednisolone 5mg OD
☐ C Increase dose of Fostair to 3 puffs BD
☐ D Stop Fostair and switch to clenil
☐ E Stop Fostair and switch to seretide 250 evohaler

85 Mr GV (72-years-old) is a known patient to the respiratory team due to his COPD. He is currently prescribed salbutamol 100mcg inhaled PRN, trimbow inhaler 1 puff OD and uniphyllin continus 400mg BD. He has been admitted to hospital due to an infective exacerbation of COPD and he has been managed accordingly with a plan to discharge tomorrow. You are the hospital pharmacist and are planning Mr GV's discharge. He informs you that he has stopped smoking whilst in hospital and is planning to remain like this for the foreseeable future. Which of the following is a CORRECT statement regarding management?

☐ A Decrease dose of uniphyllin continus after checking levels (stopping smoking)

☐ B Increase dose of uniphyllin continus after checking levels (stopping smoking)

☐ C Increase dose of trimbow due to interaction (stopping smoking)

☐ D Refer to primary care smoking cessation advisor

☐ E No intervention needed currently

86 Mr BV (65-years-old) is admitted onto the respiratory ward due to an infective exacerbation of COPD. You are the hospital pharmacist working on the respiratory ward. Mr BV's COPD medication is the following: tiotropium 18mcg inh OD, seretide 500 accuhaler 1 puff BD, salbutamol 100mcg inhaler 1-2 puffs PRN and salbutamol 2.5mg nebules inh 1 up to qds prn. The consultant has decided to initiate aminophylline therapy due to an inadequate response to bronchodilator therapy. Which of the following would be a safe range for satisfactory bronchodilation (drug levels)?

☐ A 1-10mg/Litre

☐ B 10-25mg/Litre

☐ C 10-20mg/Litre

☐ D 15-25mg/Litre

☐ E 25-100mg/Litre

87 You are a prescribing pharmacist working within primary care. Mr QT (34-years-old) has been initiated on methotrexate therapy for his rheumatoid arthritis. Mr QT has been stabilised at a dose of 15mg PO once weekly by the consultant. The consultant writes to your practice asking for you to take over the prescribing of this medication as Mr QT is now stable. Which of the following is a CORRECT statement regarding the monitoring for Mr QT?

☐ A Full blood count and renal and liver function tests every 1-2 weeks for 1 month, then every 3 months

☐ B Full blood count and renal and liver function tests every 3 months

☐ C Full blood count and renal and thyroid function tests every 1-2 weeks for 1 month, then every 3 months

☐ D Full blood count and renal and thyroid function tests every 3 months

☐ E Yearly full blood count, renal, liver and thyroid function tests as patient is now stable on the dose

88 Mr BP (aged 62-years-old) is admitted into hospital due to arrhythmias. Due to various treatments not working in the past, the consultant decides to initiate amiodarone (loading dose 200mg TDS PO for 1 week). Which of the following is a CORRECT statement regarding baseline testing?

☐ A Chest x-ray, potassium levels, liver function tests, and thyroid function tests

☐ B Chest x-ray, sodium levels, liver function tests and thyroid function tests

☐ C ECG, potassium levels, chest x-ray and thyroid function tests

☐ D ECG, sodium levels, chest x-ray and thyroid function tests

☐ E Potassium levels, liver function tests, kidney function and BP

89 Mr BG (63-years-old) will be starting chemotherapy and radiotherapy for pancreatic cancer. The consultant will be initiating him on medication to prevent hyperuricaemia. Which of the following will be the most likely medication?

☐ A Allopurinol

☐ B Docetaxel

☐ C Paclitaxel

☐ D Prednisolone

☐ E Zoledronic acid

90 Miss KC (age 33 years) is admitted onto the acute surgical admission ward due to appendicitis. She is due to be nil by mouth. You are the hospital-based pharmacist and have been asked to switch her regular medication to IV. During the medicines reconciliation, you note that she is taking phenytoin sodium capsules at 200mg PO BD. Which of the following statements is correct about her phenytoin dose?

☐ A 100mg of phenytoin sodium is approximately equivalent to 92mg phenytoin base

☐ B Miss KC does not need to remain on the same oral brand when she reverts back to oral

☐ C The usual plasma concentration for response is 10-40mg/litre

☐ D There is a low risk of congenital malformations if Miss KC were pregnant

☐ E When calculating the IV dose, the oral dose will need to be reduced by 50% due to bioavailability

91 Mr HS is attending your anticoagulation clinic due to initiation of rivaroxaban therapy. His Chads2vasc2 score is 4. What dose of rivaroxaban (if indicated) should you provide for Mr HS, who is 72-years-old, 1.8m tall, weighs 95kg, and serum creatinine is 340umol/L? You have access to the SPC: https://www.medicines.org.uk/emc/product/2793/smpc#

☐ A 10mg once daily
☐ B 15mg once daily
☐ C 15mg twice daily
☐ D 20mg once daily
☐ E Should not prescribe as not indicated

92 Mr FH (56-years-old) is admitted into hospital due to recurrent nausea, vomiting and chest pain. You are a hospital pharmacist and are completing medicines reconciliation on admission. You note Mr FH was taking digoxin 125micrograms OD PO on admission. Which of the following statements is CORRECT regarding digoxin?

☐ A For plasma digoxin levels, bloods should be taken 6 hours after the dose
☐ B Rapid intravenous use is usually recommended
☐ C Routine drug level monitoring is recommended
☐ D The dose of this medication needs to be increased by approximately 50% when co-prescribed with amiodarone
☐ E This medication is not indicated for the treatment of heart failure

93 Mr FB (48-years-old) visits your community pharmacy and is requesting another over the counter sale of ibuprofen 400mg tablets up to TDS for his back pain. He is a known patient to you and has a history of hypertension. He currently takes indapamide 2.5mg PO OD. His last BP check was 145/95. Which of the following statements is CORRECT regarding this supply?

☐ A Avoid NSAIDs in this patient due to risk factors
☐ B Avoid NSAIDs in this patient due to risk of rebound hypotension
☐ C Ibuprofen can be supplied as patients' blood pressure is well controlled
☐ D Ibuprofen can be supplied safely as patient has had this before
☐ E Ibuprofen cannot be supplied due to interaction with indapamide

94 Mr ML (74-years-old) is a diabetic patient. You are a prescribing pharmacist working in primary care and you have been asked to initiate dapagliflozin 10mg OD as therapy alongside metformin and gliclazide. Which out of the following statements is needed when counselling Mr ML on his new medication?

☐ A Report any symptoms of depression
☐ B Report any symptoms of diabetic ketoacidosis
☐ C Report any symptoms of heart failure
☐ D Report any symptoms of visual disturbances
☐ E Report any symptoms of weight gain

95 Mr BC (58-years-old) attends for his INR review at the anticoagulation clinic. You are a hospital pharmacist working with warfarin patients. Mr BC returns after four weeks and informs you he has just returned from his holiday. He enjoyed his week away in Spain and had an increased intake of green salads, leafy vegetables and various wines. He usually takes warfarin for non-valvular AF, his usual dose is 3mg OD and his INR target is 2-3. He has been taking this medication for many years (15 years) and usually within range. You action the finger prick test and todays INR reading is 3.7. There are no changes to his regular medication, no bruising or bleeding and Mr BC states he feels well in himself. He has returned to his usual lifestyle (works as an account manager) and diet/alcohol has returned to normal. What is the most appropriate action to take?

☐ A Admit to A&E due to raised INR
☐ B Omit warfarin for 2 days then return to 3mg OD dose
☐ C No changes needed
☐ D Stop taking warfarin for 1 week then recommence 3mg OD dose and return to clinic to recheck INR
☐ E Stop taking warfarin for 2 weeks then recommence 3mg OD dose for 3 days then return to clinic to check INR

96 Master YN (6 months) presents to your prescribing clinic at a walk in centre with a lump on his left arm. Mum informs you that the lump has developed where his BCG vaccine was undertaken. Master YN's image shown below:

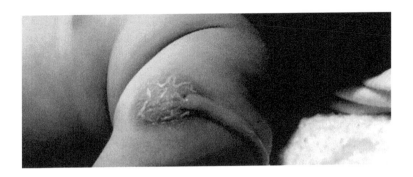

She informs you he seems to be in pain and has a temperature of 38.1. You observe all other parameters and all are in range. He is eating and drinking as normal. What is the most appropriate course of action?

- [ ] A Advise mum to apply hot, compression on the area. Keep it clean and dry. Avoid contact with any allergens/triggers. Review again in 7 days.
- [ ] B Course of antibiotics, e.g. flucloxacillin as this is potentially an infected boil and also hot, compression on the area.
- [ ] C Course of steroid needed, e.g. prednisolone as this is potentially a boil
- [ ] D No intervention needed
- [ ] E Refer to A&E

97 Miss KC (32-years-old) is reviewed by her GP for back pain. Paracetamol and naproxen have not been sufficient in management of the pain. The GP has decided to initiate Miss KC on tramadol 50mg 1 QDS PRN. You are the pharmacist who works in primary care at this surgery and also the community pharmacy based in the surgery. The GP has asked you to counsel Miss KC on her new medication. Miss KC's current medication is fluoxetine 40mg OD, salbutamol 100mcg inh PRN, desogestrel 75micrograms OD. Which of the following is a correct statement regarding the counselling?

- [ ] A Advise only to take tramadol as and when, continue with regular paracetamol
- [ ] B Advise only to take tramadol as and when, continue with regular paracetamol and NSAID
- [ ] C Advise the GP to recommend an alternative to fluoxetine

□ D Advise the GP to recommend an alternative to tramadol

□ E Explain that this is an addictive drug and should not have been prescribed

98 Miss SN (29-years-old) is on the early pregnancy admissions unit following a scan to confirm pregnancy. She is 7 weeks pregnant and soon to be discharged. You are the hospital pharmacist processing her discharge medication and she would like to discuss the use of opioids in pregnancy. She has heard about dihydrocodeine being used for pain relief (for back pain and during labour). Which of the following is the most appropriate advice to give Miss SN?

□ A Dihydrocodeine can be used during labour in pregnancy

□ B Dihydrocodeine is not safe to use in pregnancy

□ C Respiratory depression does not occur in the neonate if used during labour/delivery

□ D Side effects include hallucinations, confusion and diarrhoea

□ E There is no risk of addiction when taking this medication

99 Miss FV (24-year-old) is a regular patient at your community pharmacy. Her regular medication includes sodium valproate (for her epilepsy). She informs you in the consultation room that she is planning on becoming pregnant soon with her regular partner. Which of the following is a CORRECT statement?

□ A Refer patient to specialist to discuss risks versus benefits

□ B Remind patient of risks and refer to GP to discuss reducing dose of sodium valproate

□ C Remind patient of risks and refer to sexual health clinic due to STI risk

□ D Remind patient of risks, not to try to conceive until discussing with specialist

□ E No intervention needed, patient is discussing this with you in private and this would breach confidentiality

100 Miss LC (45-years-old) is initiated on methotrexate subcutaneous therapy for her psoriasis. She will be injecting 5 micrograms once weekly (Wednesdays). Which of the following is a CORRECT statement regarding folic acid therapy?

☐ A Folic acid 5mg to be taken once daily (apart from Wednesdays)

☐ B Folic acid 5mg to be taken once daily (on Wednesdays)

☐ C Folic acid 400 micrograms to be taken once daily (apart from Wednesdays)

☐ D Folic acid 400 micrograms to be taken once weekly

☐ E Folic acid only recommended when patients take methotrexate orally

Medium weighted questions

101 Miss SY, a 24-year-old Caucasian woman with no medical history, comes into the community pharmacy requesting the morning after pill. She advises that she was hesitant to come in due to a fear of stigma associated with unprotected sexual intercourse. She is unsure whether she can obtain the morning after pill since it has been just under 5 days since it took place. She advises that her last menstrual period was 2 weeks ago. Which is the most appropriate management for this patient?

☐A Desogestrel 75mg daily for 28 days

☐B Insert copper IUD

☐C Patient should be referred to GP since the time for any emergency contraception to take effect has lapsed

☐D Take levonorgestrel 1.5mg stat

☐E Take urlipristal 30mg stat

102 Miss BA, a 31-year-old Caucasian woman, has recently given birth and is currently breastfeeding. She complains of white vaginal discharge with a pungent fish smell; the doctor confirms it is bacterial vaginosis. What is the most appropriate and cost-effective treatment for this patient?

☐A Clindamycin 2% vaginal cream – use nightly for 7 nights

☐B Clotrimazole 2% cream – use two - three times a day

☐C Metronidazole 0.75% vaginal gel – use nightly for 5 nights

☐D Metronidazole 2g PO STAT

☐E Metronidazole 400mg PO BD for 7 days

103 Miss JS, a 24-year-old female, wants to start on the combined hormonal contraceptive pill as she has done some reading and feels this is the most appropriate option for her. She visits your community pharmacy to discuss possible options. In what case would it be contraindicated for this patient?

- ☐ A BMI of 30
- ☐ B BP 163/101
- ☐ C Current smoker
- ☐ D Family history of venous thromboembolism
- ☐ E Uncomplication organ transplant

104 Miss SL, a 25-year-old Caucasian woman, is currently on phenytoin for her epilepsy. You are a prescribing pharmacist in an outpatient hospital pharmacy. The neurologist wants to keep her on phenytoin and asks that you prescribe her contraception as she is aware of the pregnancy risks associated with taking phenytoin. Miss SL doesn't want to fall pregnant but is currently sexually active. Which of the methods of contraception is most appropriate for this patient?

- ☐ A Combined hormonal contraception
- ☐ B Levonogestrel–releasing intrauterine device
- ☐ C Progesterone-only-implant
- ☐ D Progesterone-only-pill
- ☐ E Urlipristal emergency contraception

105 Mr EM, a 49-year-old Caucasian man, presents to the community pharmacy complaining of erectile dysfunction. He wants to know more about this condition and what causes it. What statement is FALSE regarding erectile dysfunction?

- ☐ A All men with unexplained erectile dysfunction should be evaluated for the presence of cardiovascular risk factors and any identified risk should be addressed.
- ☐ B Erectile dysfunction can occur as a side-effect of drugs such as antihypertensives, antidepressants, antipsychotics, cytotoxic drugs and recreational drugs (including alcohol).
- ☐ C Erectile dysfunction increases the risk of cardiovascular disease.
- ☐ D Oral phosphodiesterase type-5 inhibitor is the first line drug treatment and acts by initiating an erection.
- ☐ E The recommended approach for management of erectile dysfunction is a combination of drug treatment and lifestyle changes.

106 Prolonged use of proton pump inhibitors (PPI) greater than a year can cause:

☐ **A** Hyperkalaemia
☐ **B** Hypermagnesemia
☐ **C** Hypernatraemia
☐ **D** Hypokalaemia
☐ **E** Hypomagnesaemia

107 Mr SH, a 47-year-old Caucasian man, has been advised to visit the community pharmacy to purchase some laxatives; his GP has informed him that it is likely being caused by the morphine he is taking. Which laxative should be avoided in this patient?

☐ **A** Bisacodyl
☐ **B** Docusate
☐ **C** Ispaghula husk
☐ **D** Lactulose
☐ **E** Senna

108 You are a clinical pharmacist working in a minor illness setting in primary care. Mrs AA, a 38-year-old Asian woman, attends your practice advising she is experiencing 'irritable bowel syndrome symptoms'. Which symptom listed below is not typical of IBS?

☐ **A** Bloating
☐ **B** Constipation
☐ **C** Diarrhoea
☐ **D** Stomach cramps
☐ **E** Vomiting

109 Mrs FG (38-years-old) visits your community pharmacy and presents for a prescription requesting orlistat. In which circumstance is orlistat NOT suitable for prescribing?

☐ **A** A patient with a BMI of 26 who is diagnosed with type 2 diabetes
☐ **B** A patient with a BMI of 29 who is diagnosed with hypertension and depression

☐ C A patient with a BMI of 30

☐ D A patient with a BMI of 32 who is diagnosed with hypercholesterolaemia and gastritis

☐ E A patient with a BMI of 40

110 You have been asked to counsel a patient on the management for diverticular disease. Which statement is TRUE with regards to the management of diverticular disease?

☐ A Antibiotics are not recommended for patients with diverticular disease

☐ B Avoid simple analgesia such as paracetamol in patients with ongoing abdominal pain

☐ C Bulk forming laxatives should not be considered when a high-fibre diet is unsuitable or for patients with persistent constipation or diarrhoea

☐ D NSAID and opioid analgesics are recommended

☐ E Patients with diverticulosis or diverticular disease should be advised to avoid whole grains, fruits and vegetables

111 Mrs JF (age 32 years) has recently been initiated on salbutamol inhaled therapy for asthma management. She has been advised that this is an example of a selective beta-2 agonist. Which adverse effect can be caused by using selective beta-2 agonists?

☐ A Hypercalcaemia

☐ B Hyperkalaemia

☐ C Hypernatraemia

☐ D Hypokalaemia

☐ E Hyponatraemia

112 Mr SA, a 52-year-old man, comes into your prescribing clinic (at the GP surgery) for a post discharge COPD review. You note that he is currently using a salbutamol inhaler; he informs you that he uses two puffs up to four times a day whenever he needs it. Recently it seems that he is using it more often. He was admitted into hospital over a week ago because of his breathing. Since discharge he has been feeling more breathless than

usual, however he does not feel unwell. You undertake a spirometry test and find that his FEV1 is less than 50%; his FBC reveals an eosinophil level of 0.2/L. What is the most appropriate management for this patient given his symptoms and the results?

☐ A Add in incruse ellipta inhaler
☐ B Add in relvar ellipta 92/22 micrograms inhaler
☐ C Add in trelegy ellipta DPI inhaler
☐ D No changes needed
☐ E Patient to attend A&E due to eosinophil level

113 Mrs LK (58-years-old) has been prescribed clarithromycin 500mg tablets ONE twice a day for 5 days for her infective COPD exacerbation. You are a hospital pharmacist working on the acute respiratory ward and you notice she is on a medication that needs to be withheld whilst she takes the course of clarithromycin. Which of the following medications needs to be withheld?

☐ A Amlodipine
☐ B Carvediol
☐ C Gabapentin
☐ D Relvar ellipta
☐ E Simvastatin

114 Mr HL (68-years-old) is currently prescribed uniphyllin continus 200mg tablets for his chronic asthma. What is the therapeutic drug range for his medication?

☐ A 0 – 5mg/L
☐ B 10 – 20mg/L
☐ C 15 – 25mg/L
☐ D 20 – 35mg/L
☐ E 30 – 45mg/L

115 Mr GV (58-years-old) visits your community pharmacy requesting an emergency supply of his salbutamol inhaler. He informs you that in the last 3 days his asthma has been uncontrolled, and he has been using his

blue inhaler over 10 times per day. He is struggling to cope at home. When would a patient be considered as having near-fatal acute asthma attack?

☐ A Cyanosis
☐ B Heart Rate greater than or equal to 110/min
☐ C Inability to complete sentences in one breath
☐ D Peak flow <33% best or predicted
☐ E Raised $PaCO_2$ and/or the need for mechanical ventilation with raised inflation pressures

116 Mrs JO (28-years-old) attends your chronic disease management clinic within primary care. She presents with symptoms of lethargy, pallor and irritability. You book her in for a blood test and note that she has low vitamin B12 levels. What is the likely diagnosis for this patient?

☐ A Aplastic anaemia
☐ B Haemolytic anaemia
☐ C Iron deficiency anaemia
☐ D Megaloblastic anaemia
☐ E Sickle cell anaemia

For questions 117-120

Using the most appropriate word in the list below, complete the table to match the electrolyte imbalance with the most appropriate treatment. Note all cases listed below are for patients where the electrolyte imbalance is of a mild to moderate nature.

- Hyperkalaemia
- Hypernatraemia
- Hyperphosphataemia
- Hypocalcaemia
- Hypomagnesaemia
- Hypophosphataemia
- Slow sodium

	Electrolyte imbalance	Treatment
117		Calcium resonium®
118	Hyponatraemia	
119		Sandocal 1000® effervescent tablets
120		Phosphate Sandoz® effervescent tablet

121 A 56-year-old woman describes symptoms of hot flushes, particularly at night, which are accompanied with sleep disturbances and low mood. She is also experiencing 'brain fog', low libido and menstrual irregularities. Her GP has diagnosed her with menopause and prescribed a trial of oestrogel and utrogestan for 12 days of the month with a plan to review after 3 months. She presents to your community pharmacy and queries whether she should still be taking her regular contraception. Which of the following is the most APPROPRIATE advice?

☐ A   No, she does not need contraception.
☐ B   No, she does not need contraception because this will be provided by the oestrogel and utrogestan.
☐ C   Yes, she still needs contraception because she is still menstruating.
☐ D   Yes, she still needs contraception because she is still sexually active.
☐ E   Yes, she still needs contraception but only barrier methods.

122 Mrs BF (aged 59-years-old) has been prescribed mirabegron 25mg OD after no success with three different antimuscarinics for her overactive bladder. Which one of the following is important to monitor before initiation of mirabegron?

☐ A   Blood pressure
☐ B   Creatinine clearance
☐ C   Liver function tests (LFT)s
☐ D   Pulse
☐ E   Urea and electrolytes

123 You are a prescribing pharmacist within primary care. A 67-year-old man reports an increase in urinary frequency and urgency. He has noticed blood on passing urine and has recently been experiencing symptoms of erectile dysfunction. He has handed in a urine sample which has returned

as normal from microbiology cultures. After a discussion with the GP regarding his symptoms, what is the most appropriate next step?

☐ A Blood test to check HbA1C
☐ B Rectal examination
☐ C Rectal examination and PSA blood test
☐ D Routine referral to specialist (urology)
☐ E Urgent 2 week referral to specialist (urology)

124 Mr SH (73-years-old) was diagnosed with a hiatus hernia via an endoscopy 7 years ago. He was prescribed omeprazole 20mg BD PO and has continued on this dose since. He informs you his symptoms are well managed. Recently however, he has been feeling exceptionally tired, dizzy and light headed when standing up from a sitting position. Which one of the following is most likely the cause of his current symptoms as a result of long-term PPI use?

☐ A Exacerbation reflux symptoms caused by the hiatus hernia
☐ B Folate deficiency
☐ C Iron deficiency anaemia
☐ D Urea and electrolyte disturbances
☐ E Vitamin B12 deficiency

125 Mrs HK (34-years-old) is diagnosed with ulcerative colitis following a raised faecal calprotectin result and review by the gastroenterology team at her local hospital. A colonoscopy is undertaken to review her condition. What would they have seen on the imaging for this diagnosis?

☐ A Continuous full thickness from the mouth to the anus
☐ B Full thickness from the mouth to the anus but not continuous
☐ C Full thickness inflammation in the oesophagus
☐ D Inflammation and continuous partial thickness in the rectum that extends through the colon
☐ E Partial thickness and inflammation in the oesophagus with fistulae and/or abscesses

126 You are conducting an annual medication review for a 68-year-old man with diagnosed COPD. In order to check his understanding, you ask

him to show you how he uses his inhalers. He is currently prescribed the Fostair 100/6 inhaler for prevention. What is the CORRECT description for how this should be used?

☐ A For the salbutamol: shake the inhaler, take the cap off and breathe out gently to empty the lungs. Put your lips around the mouthpiece, start to breathe in slowly and steadily and at the same time press the cannister down once. Continue to breathe in slowly until your lungs feel full, then hold for 10 seconds, or as long as comfortable, and leave at least 30 seconds between a second dose. Repeat the above for the Fostair but breathe in quickly and deeply.

☐ B Shake the inhaler, take the cap off and breathe out gently to empty the lungs. Put your lips around the mouthpiece, start to breathe in slowly and steadily and at the same time press the cannister down once. Continue to breathe in slowly until your lungs feel full, then hold for 10 seconds, or as long as comfortable, and leave at least 30 seconds between a second dose.

☐ C Shake the inhaler, take the cap off and breathe out gently to empty the lungs. Put your lips around the mouthpiece, start to breathe in slowly and steadily and at the same time press the cannister down once. Continue to breathe in slowly until your lungs feel full, then hold for 30 seconds, or as long as comfortable, and leave at least 1 minute between a second dose.

☐ D Shake the inhaler, take the cap off and put your lips around the mouthpiece. Press the cannister down once and then start to breathe in slowly and steadily. Continue to breathe in slowly until your lungs feel full, then hold for 10 seconds, or as long as comfortable, and leave at least 30 seconds between a second dose.

☐ E Shake the inhaler, take the cap off and put your lips around the mouthpiece. Start to breathe in quickly and deeply and at the same time press the cannister down once. Continue to breathe in slowly until your lungs feel full, then hold for 10 seconds, or as long as comfortable, and leave at least 30 seconds between a second dose.

127 Master JK (4-years-old) is prescribed long term clenil 50mcg evohaler 1puff BD and salbutamol 2 puffs PRN for his childhood asthma. Which of the following are essential long term monitoring for this patient?

☐ A Chest examination 6 monthly
☐ B Full blood count annually
☐ C Height and weight 6 monthly
☐ D Height and weight annually
☐ E Serum potassium annually

128 Mr GN (42-years-old) has been admitted to hospital and diagnosed with chronic alcoholism. You are a hospital pharmacist working on acute admissions. The consultant informs you that Mr GN is at risk of Wernicke's encephalopathy and Korsakoff's psychosis and should be prescribed a vitamin to help reduce this risk. Which one of the following is the most APPROPRIATE drug to prescribe?

☐ A Ascorbic acid
☐ B Colecalciferol
☐ C Folic acid
☐ D Iron
☐ E Thiamine

129 Miss SB is a 28-year-old female patient that has had a recent blood test to see if her symptoms are related to a deficiency. She suffers with heavy periods as a result of her endometriosis and has recently been feeling very tired and short of breath. She mentions that she previously had this same problem and was prescribed something called ferrous sulphate that made her very constipated. What is the most appropriate advice?

☐ A Although best absorbed on an empty stomach, advise to take after food to reduce gastro-intestinal side effects
☐ B Dissolve the tablets in a glass of water
☐ C Half the usual dose that is prescribed
☐ D Take the prescribed vitamin on an empty stomach
☐ E Take the tablets on alternate days

130 A 50-year-old male has come into the community pharmacy requesting to speak to you in private. In the consultation room he explains that he has been struggling to maintain an erection for the past few months and it is starting to affect the relationship with his partner. He wondered if

there was any medication that he could use to overcome this concern. After taking a thorough medical history, you deem it appropriate to sell Viagra Connect over-the-counter. Which of the following counseling points would be LEAST appropriate to advise?

- ☐ A Contact doctor within 6 months for a clinical review
- ☐ B In order for the medication to be effective sexual stimulation is required
- ☐ C One or two 50mg tablets should be taken with water approximately one hour before anticipated sexual activity
- ☐ D Seek immediate medical assistance if painful erection lasts longer than 4 hours (priapism)
- ☐ E When taken with food the onset of activity may be delayed compared to a fasted state

131 A 25-year-old female with a BMI of 32kg/m2 has requested an emergency contraceptive following an episode of unprotected sexual intercourse 48 hours ago. You also note that the patient is taking rifampicin 900mg TDS for the treatment of tuberculosis. There are no safeguarding concerns. Which of the following would be the most appropriate form of contraception for this patient?

- ☐ A Desogestrel 75 microgram tablets
- ☐ B Intrauterine copper device
- ☐ C Levonorgestrel 1500 microgram tablet
- ☐ D Levonorgestrel 150 microgram/ethinylestradiol 30 microgram tablets
- ☐ E Ulipristal 30mg tablet

132 A 35-year-old female is due to undergo cholecystectomy, a major surgery in 2 months' time. She is currently taking a regular contraceptive that should be stopped at least 4 weeks before the procedure. Which of the following contraception is the patient likely to be taking?

- ☐ A Desogestrel 75 microgram tablets
- ☐ B Intrauterine copper device
- ☐ C Levonorgestrel 1500 microgram tablet
- ☐ D Levonorgestrel 150 microgram/ethinylestradiol 30 microgram tablets
- ☐ E Ulipristal 30mg tablet

133 A 65-year-old female with a past medical history of Crohn's disease would like to purchase a product over-the-counter for a sore throat. She tested positive for coronavirus 6 months ago but since then has fully recovered. The patient feels well in herself and takes the following medication:

- Amlodipine 10mg once daily
- Lansoprazole 15mg once daily
- Sulfasalazine 1g four times a day
- Perindopril erbumine 4mg once daily

Which of the following would be the most appropriate course of action?

☐ A Do not treat; see GP if unresolved within 7 days
☐ B Refer to accident & emergency (A&E)
☐ C Refer to GP urgently
☐ D Treat with over-the-counter medicine and provide advice on prognosis
☐ E Treat with over-the-counter medicine; see GP if unresolved within 7 days

For the scenarios described below, select the corresponding medication from the list above. Each option may be used once, more than once, or not at all.

Theme: Laxatives

☐ A Bisacodyl
☐ B Co-danthrusate
☐ C Docusate
☐ D Glycerol suppository
☐ E Ispaghula husk
☐ F Lactulose
☐ G Senna
☐ H Sodium picosulfate

134 A 90-year-old female is under palliative care; she has been constipated for the past few days due to receiving large doses of opioids in a syringe driver. The laxative prescribed for the patient by the palliative care team

is a stimulant laxative that is potentially carcinogenic according to animal studies. It can also change the colour of urine to red.

135 An 18-year-old female has been advised by her GP to purchase a stimulant laxative from a pharmacy. The GP mentioned the laxative has an onset of action of 8-12 hours and also warned that it can change the colour of urine to yellow/red-brown.

136 A 4-year-old child has been rushed into your community pharmacy after swallowing a peanut a few minutes ago. The child's face and lips have become swollen and is short of breath. You suspect the child maybe having an anaphylactic reaction. You ask a colleague to contact 999 and decide to administer adrenaline using a pre-filled pen. Which of the following strength of adrenaline would be appropriate to administer to this child?

☐ A 150micrograms, then repeated after 5–15 minutes as required
☐ B 300micrograms, then repeated after 5–15 minutes as required
☐ C 500micrograms, then repeated after 5–15 minutes as required
☐ D 150mg, then repeated after 5–15 minutes as required
☐ E 500mg, then repeated after 5–15 minutes as required

137 A 70-year-old male with a past medical history of poorly controlled asthma has been initiated uniphyllin continus (theophylline) on the advice of a respiratory consultant. The patient had a blood test 5 days after starting the new medication to ensure the dose was safe for the patient. The plasma concentration was found to be elevated despite being prescribed a low dose. You are working in the medicines information department and have been asked to identify factors that can affect the levels of theophylline. Which of the following factors would most likely increase the plasma level of theophylline?

☐ A Alcohol
☐ B Heart failure
☐ C Smoking
☐ D St John's wort
☐ E Rifampicin

138 A 23-year-old male's asthma management plan has been stepped up following an asthma review with a respiratory nurse. The nurse would like to initiate the patient on a Maintenance and Reliever Therapy (MART) regime. You are a Primary Care Network (PCN) pharmacist and have been asked to recommend a suitable inhaler. Which of the following inhalers would be suitable for MART therapy?

☐ A Atrovent (ipratropium)
☐ B Braltus (tiotropium)
☐ C Combisal (salmeterol + fluticasone)
☐ D Luforbec (formoterol + beclometasone)
☐ E Salamol (salbutamol)

For the scenarios described below, select the most appropriate supplement from the list above. Each option may be used once, more than once or not at all.

Theme: Nutritional supplements

☐ A Vitamin A
☐ B Vitamin B1
☐ C Vitamin B6
☐ D Vitamin B7
☐ E Vitamin B12
☐ F Vitamin C
☐ G Vitamin D
☐ H Vitamin K

139 A 40-year-old male patient with pernicious anaemia has been informed by his GP that he has a lack of intrinsic factor in his body to absorb a vitamin. He must now be administered this vitamin to correct any deficiencies.

140 A 32-year-old female patient requiring treatment for scurvy.

141 A 33-year-old pregnant patient who should avoid purchasing this vitamin due to the risk of high levels causing birth defects.

142 Vitamin recommended in those who may develop a deficiency, particularly individuals with dark skin (such as those of African, African-Caribbean or South Asian origin).

143 A 62-year-old patient is admitted into A&E due to excessive bleeding. This vitamin is required as part of treatment. (Medication on admission: amlodipine, levothyroxine, simvastatin and warfarin.)

For the scenarios described below, select the most appropriate option from the list above. Each option may be used once, more than once or none at all.

Theme: Adverse drug reaction

- ☐ A Hypercalcaemia
- ☐ B Hyperglycaemia
- ☐ C Hyperkalaemia
- ☐ D Hypermagnesemia
- ☐ E Hypernatraemia
- ☐ F Hypoglycaemia
- ☐ G Hyponatraemia
- ☐ H Hypomagnesaemia

144 A 65-year-old male patient has been taking omeprazole 20mg daily for the past 30 years to manage dyspepsia. His blood test shows a gradual change in an electrolyte.

145 A 78-year-old patient has been taking fluoxetine 20mg daily for the last 6 months. He has been admitted onto the acute ward due to drowsiness.

146 A 52-year-old patient with known malignancy. The drug of choice to correct abnormal levels is pamidronate.

147 A 77-year-old patient is started on bisoprolol. His current medications are: lansoprazole, metformin, glimepiride, ramipril, clopidogrel and atorvastatin. What is he at risk of developing?

148 An 80-year-old patient is initiated on spironolactone as add on to his current furesomide for known congestive heart failure. What is he at risk of developing?

For the scenarios described below, select the most appropriate cytotoxic drug from the list above. Each option may be used once, more than once, or not at all.

Theme: Cytotoxic medication

☐ A Bleomycin
☐ B Cabazitaxel
☐ C Cisplatin
☐ D Doxorubicin
☐ E Etoposide
☐ F Methotrexate
☐ G Mitomycin
☐ H Vinblastine

149 A 65-year-old male patient has a rare metastatic cancer that affects the bone marrow. You are a clinical pharmacist working on an oncology ward. An oncology specialist would like to know which cytotoxic drugs do not cause bone marrow suppression.

150 This drug is available as three different formulations: conventional, liposomal and pegylated. They all vary in their licensing and are NOT interchangeable.

151 This injection is for intravenous administration only. Inadvertent intrathecal administration can cause severe neurotoxicity, which is usually fatal.

152 Miss JH (33-years-old) is initiated on this medication for her rheumatoid arthritis. The consultant in secondary care initiates but after dose stabilising – the care of medication is given to the primary care clinicians. Miss JH is now stable on this medication and requires regular blood test monitoring.

153 A 35-year-old female patient has been prescribed a medication for the management of an autoimmune condition. She has been advised to use effective contraception during treatment and for at least 6 months after the treatment ends. Which of the following medication is likely to have been prescribed?

☐ A Azathioprine
☐ B Methotrexate
☐ C Mycophenolate
☐ D Sulfasalazine
☐ E Tacrolimus

154 You are a practice pharmacist conducting a medication safety on non-steroid anti-inflammatory drugs (NSAIDs) due to their risk of gastrointestinal bleeding. Your audit consists of reviewing if there is adequate gastroprotection for those taking NSAID long term. In order to prioritise your workload you intend to search by NSAIDs that have the highest risk, then work down to the those of a lower risk. Which of the following NSAIDs poses the highest risk of a gastrointestinal bleed?

☐ A Celecoxib
☐ B Diclofenac
☐ C Ibuprofen
☐ D Indometacin
☐ E Piroxicam

155 Mr JW, a 57-year-old man, attends your community pharmacy for advice. He gives a history of being unable to attain an erection despite sexual stimulation. On questioning, Mr JW tells you he is a data analyst and works at a desk for his full-time job. He takes part in minimal exercise and smokes 20 cigarettes a day. You check Mr JW's height and weight: he is 1.82m tall and weighs 109kg. Which of the following are correct?

☐ A A phosphodiesterase type-5 inhibitor could be prescribed
☐ B Mr JW's BMI shows he is obese
☐ C Mr JW is at higher risk of cardiovascular disease
☐ D Sildenafil should be avoided in severe hepatic impairment
☐ E All of the above

156 Mrs TW, a 35-year-old female, attends your community pharmacy with a prescription for microgynon 30. You check her patient medical record and she has not had this before. The PMR does show that Mrs TW is also on: salbutamol inhaler 2 puffs inh qds prn, clenil modulite 50mcg inhaler

1 puff inh bd, carbamazepine 200mg PO tds. Which of the following statements is CORRECT?

- [ ] A Carbamazepine is an enzyme inhibitor
- [ ] B Mrs TW can safely continue to take microgynon if she stops the carbamazepine
- [ ] C Mrs TW should be advised to explore alternative contraceptive methods
- [ ] D The dose of carbamazepine indicates she has epilepsy
- [ ] E The effectiveness of microgynon is unaffected by carbamazepine

157 Which of these following statements about hormonal therapy is FALSE?

- [ ] A Clonidine is a useful option for patients requiring HRT who also experience hot flushing.
- [ ] B If a patient forgets to take their Moonia pill and remembers within 3 hours of the usual time of taking, they can take their missed pill without experiencing a reduction in efficacy.
- [ ] C Patients with intact uterus wishing to use HRT should be given a combined oestrogen and progesterone therapy.
- [ ] D Taking a CHC with no hormone-free interval is a licenced regimen, useful for patients with heavy or painful withdrawal bleeds.
- [ ] E The effectiveness of combined hormonal contraception can be reduced by enzyme inducing drugs.

158 Miss LS, a 32-year-old woman, has been booked into your surgery clinic. You are an independent prescriber working within your remit of women's health. She provides a history of grey discharge that has a distinct fishy smell. She has tried a vaginal soap to get rid of the smell, but it hasn't improved and actually has got worse. She has no itching or soreness. Miss LS has 1 long-term sexual partner, has no children, and is not pregnant. She has had no recent medical history of note. Miss LS does explain that she is planning to attend her hen-do in 2 days' time and is expecting to have a few alcoholic drinks. How do you proceed?

- [ ] A Advise Miss LS to use a vaginal douche
- [ ] B Prescribe intravaginal metronidazole gel 0.75% once daily for 5 days

    ☐ **C** Prescribe oral metronidazole 400mg bd for 5 days
    ☐ **D** Refer to colleague for vulval examination
    ☐ **E** Refer to GUM clinic

159 Miss GR (age 23-years-old) presents to your community pharmacy asking for emergency contraception. On questioning, she tells you she had unprotected sexual intercourse 4 days ago. You check your PMR and find she had a prescription for Cerelle dispensed two weeks ago. She has been delayed starting this prescription and has not had any hormonal contraception for 3 weeks. Which of the following statements is false?

    ☐ **A** A copper intrauterine contraceptive device may be offered
    ☐ **B** Miss GR should start taking her Cerelle tablets immediately
    ☐ **C** Miss GR should use condoms or abstain from sexual intercourse
    ☐ **D** Ulipristal is a suitable option for emergency contraception
    ☐ **E** None of the above

160 Mr MO, a 43-year-old male, comes into your community pharmacy asking for advice on the heartburn he's been experiencing for the last 2 weeks. He describes a feeling of burning pain at the base of his throat, worse at night. He has tried lifting the head of the bed with extra pillows, but this has not helped. His current medication is ramipril 10mg daily for hypertension, citalopram 20mg daily for stress-related anxiety, atorvastatin 40mg at night due to QRISK of 37%. Mr MO has also been buying ibuprofen 400mg for back pain over the last 2 months. Which of the following statements is CORRECT?

    ☐ **A** Barrett's oesophagus is a form of cancer caused by excessive acid in the base of the oesophagus
    ☐ **B** Gaviscon may be used long-term for the symptoms of dyspepsia
    ☐ **C** Lansoprazole 30mg daily should be offered to any patient with more than 2 risk factors for developing dyspepsia
    ☐ **D** Patients must stop their proton pump inhibitor for 4 weeks before undertaking urea (13C) breath test for *Helicobacter pylori* infection
    ☐ **E** None of the above

For the following 5 questions (161-165), choose the best answer:

☐ A Blackened stools
☐ B Constipation
☐ C Diarrhoea
☐ D Dyspepsia
☐ E All of the above

161 Can be a symptom of Crohn's disease and eased by colestyramine?

162 Can be a symptom of *C. difficile* infection, particularly if the patient is also taking a PPI and/or recently taken a course of antibiotics?

163 Is a common side-effect of iron therapy?

164 Can be treated with prucalopride when other options have failed to produce an adequate response?

165 Can be a symptom of stomach cancer?

166 Mr FS, a 14-year-old male, has been booked into your surgery clinic. You are a prescribing pharmacist who manages respiratory patients. Mr FS has been refused a repeat request for a salbutamol inhaler after reaching his maximum count of allowed prescriptions. Mr FS has used 10 ventolin inhalers in the last 12 months. On questioning, he describes needing to use his ventolin inhaler almost every day. He enjoys playing football but finds he needs to stop due to breathlessness; this is affecting his mood and he is getting very frustrated with himself. He is also prescribed a clenil inhaler 200mcg and uses 2 puffs twice daily. What is the next APPROPRIATE step?

☐ A Change to Symbicort 100/6 turbohaler 1 puff twice daily and 1 puff as required for relief of symptoms, increased if necessary up to 6 puffs as required, max. 8 puffs per day
☐ B Change to Symbicort 100/6 turbohaler 2 puffs bd
☐ C Check inhaler technique
☐ D Co-prescribe montelukast 5mg at night
☐ E Increase clenil inhaler to 400mcg bd

167 Mrs LR, a 39-year-old female, is due for her annual medication review. She has had an asthma review with the nurse which states the following:

Asthma - Adult

Review

Review: Attended clinic for annual Asthma review. Asthma seems well controlled at the moment and patient not having to use SABA any more then 1-2 times per months. No changes made today advised to continue with current treatment. Fostair 2 puffs BD and SABA PRN.

Smoking cessation advice given – social smoker

Asthma causes daytime symptoms 1 to 2 times per month

Asthma never causes night symptoms

Asthma not limiting activities

Asthma trigger - perfume

Asthma trigger - animals

ICS use: Using inhaled steroids - low dose

Bronchodilator used infrequently

Number of exacerbations in past year: 0

PEFR: 550 L/min

Asthma - currently active

Inhaler compliance: Good compliance with inhaler

Inhaler technique: Inhaler technique - good

Rescue meds: Treatment not indicated

Influenza immunisation advised: Yes given today

Mrs LR is currently prescribed Fostair 200/6 inhaler 2 puffs bd and ventolin evohaler 1-2 puffs prn for breathlessness. What is the next APPROPRIATE step?

☐ A Advise Mrs LR that she should continue with her prescribed treatment and stop smoking

☐ B Change the Fostair inhaler to a clenil 100mcg inhaler 1 puff bd

☐ C Change the Fostair inhaler to a clenil 100mcg inhaler 2 puffs bd

☐ D Stop the Fostair inhaler and continue on ventolin prn

☐ E Suggest that Mrs LR could reduce her Fostair to 1 puff bd

168 Your patient has COPD and is attending your respiratory clinic today for review of their treatment. They are currently taking anoro ellipta 1 puff once daily, ventolin evohaler 1-2 puffs QDS prn and seretide evohaler 125mcg 1 puff bd. Which statement is FALSE?

- □ A The patient is receiving duplication of therapy which requires optimisation
- □ B The patient may have had >2 moderate exacerbations in the previous year
- □ C The patient may have some asthma/COPD crossover features
- □ D The patient may require a spacer device
- □ E This patient is not indicated for pneumococcal vaccine

169 You are an independent prescriber working competently within respiratory at your local acute hospital. You have been asked to provide a training session to newly qualified nurses. Which statement is TRUE of the management of COPD?

- □ A All spacers are interchangeable with all MDI devices
- □ B Azithromycin is licenced as prophylactic therapy to reduce the risk of acute exacerbations
- □ C Oral mucolytics may be prescribed to prevent exacerbations in people with stable COPD
- □ D Roflumilast is a phosphodiesterase type-5 inhibitor with anti-inflammatory properties
- □ E None of the above

170 You are a community pharmacist and are currently helping support a pre-registration pharmacist understand medication. Consider the following statements about antihistamines. Which statement is TRUE regarding fexofenadine?

- □ A Is not suitable for a patient advised to take a low sodium diet
- □ B May be given to a child aged 8-years-old at a dose of 60mg daily
- □ C Penetrates the blood brain barrier to a greater extent than promethazine
- □ D Requires warning label 2 to be added to dispensing labels
- □ E Should not be given with promethazine due to the increased exposure to fexofenadine

For each of the following conditions/scenarios, choose the best course of treatment and follow-up:

171 Pernicious anaemia – most APPROPRIATE treatment?

- ☐ A Cyanocobalamin 100mcg daily with annual B12 level
- ☐ B Cyanocobalamin 150mcg daily
- ☐ C Hydroxocobalamin 1mg 3-monthly I/M
- ☐ D Hydroxocobalamin 1mg 3-monthly I/M lifelong with annual b12 level
- ☐ E Hydroxocobalamin I/M; initially 1mg 3 times a week for 2 weeks, then 1mg every 3 months

172 Folate rescue therapy whilst taking methotrexate

- ☐ A Folic acid 400mcg daily except on day of methotrexate dose
- ☐ B Folic acid 5mg daily except on day of methotrexate dose
- ☐ C Folic acid 5mg weekly, on a different day to the methotrexate dose
- ☐ D Folic acid 5mg weekly, on the same day as the methotrexate dose
- ☐ E Folic acid 400mg weekly, on a different day to the methotrexate dose

173 Prevention of neural tube defects in an adult trying to conceive who has previously had a child with spina bifida.

- ☐ A 400mcg daily started before conception for the duration of the pregnancy
- ☐ B 400mcg daily started before conception until week 12 of pregnancy
- ☐ C 5mg daily started before conception for the duration of the pregnancy
- ☐ D 5mg daily started before conception until week 12 of pregnancy
- ☐ E As per consultant recommendation

174 Confirmed cow's milk allergy in a breastfed baby.

- ☐ A Stop breastfeeding and prescribe Aptamil Pepti 1 until child is 1 year
- ☐ B Stop breastfeeding and prescribe SMA Alfamino until child is weaned
- ☐ C Stop breastfeeding and prescribe SMA Wysoy until child is 1 year
- ☐ D Support the breast-feeding parent to eliminate all cow's milk from their diet and prescribe calcium and vitamin D supplementation
- ☐ E Support the continuation of breast-feeding and prescribe Neocate Syneo to supplement diet

175 A patient taking azathioprine with the following blood monitoring results:

Haemoglobin concentration 129 g/dL (115-160)

Mean cell volume 88 fL (79-97)

Total White Blood Count 0.52 x10⁹/L (4-10)

Neutrophils 2.5 x 10⁹/L (1.8-10)

Platelets 108 x10⁹/L (140-450)

☐ A Continue treatment and repeat blood test

☐ B Continue treatment at a lower dose, bloods in 3 months

☐ C Continue treatment with no change, bloods in 3 months

☐ D Stop treatment and contact specialty department for advice

☐ E Withhold treatment for 1 week and then continue as before, bloods in 1 month

Low Weighted Questions

For questions 176-179.

For the scenarios described below, select the single most likely treatment from the list above. Each option may be used once, more than one or not at all.

Theme – Drugs initiated in secondary care

☐ A Azathioprine
☐ B Bicalutamide
☐ C Hydrocarbamide
☐ D Methotrexate
☐ E Tacrolimus
☐ F Tamoxifen

176 Mrs LP, a 66-year-old woman, is in remission for breast cancer. She has been prescribed a drug for the primary prevention of cancer since she is considered to be moderate to high risk.

177 Mr HJ, a 58-year-old man, has been diagnosed with severe active rheumatoid arthritis and has not trialled any disease modifying drugs yet.

178 Mr WE, a 72-year-old man, who has recently been diagnosed with advanced prostate cancer; the specialist requests this treatment is prescribed alongside gonadorelin analogue.

179 Mr JO, a 42-year-old, has undergone a kidney transplantation. This treatment is a prophylaxis of graft rejection which is given 24 hours after transplantation.

180 Mr PO, a 52-year-old man, attends the minor ailments prescribing clinic with inflammation on his big toe. He informs you that he has had this pain before and was given medication for gout. On examination you confirm that it is an acute gout attack. You note he is on blood pressure medication. What is the most appropriate treatment for this patient?

☐ A Allopurinol
☐ B Colchicine
☐ C Diclofenac
☐ D Febuxostat
☐ E Paracetamol

181 Miss AP, a 22-year-old woman, attends the community pharmacy with irritation in her eye. She describes being sensitive to light, her eyes feel sore and she seems to have a redness around her iris associated with watering. You ask her whether she wears contact lenses and she informs you that she accidentally fell asleep with them on yesterday. What is the likely diagnosis based on the patient's symptoms?

☐ A Bacterial conjunctivitis
☐ B Blepharitis
☐ C Keratitis
☐ D Subconjunctival haemorrhage
☐ E Uveitis

182 Mr JK, a 39-year-old man, attends the community pharmacy complaining of dry eyes. He is requesting treatment medication. He has nil allergies and nil medical history. Which of the following is NOT used in the treatment of dry eyes?

☐ A Clinitas carbomer
☐ B Hylo-forte
☐ C Hypromellose
☐ D Lacri-lube
☐ E Maxitrol

183 Mr PJ, a 5-year-old boy, has come into the pharmacy with his mother. His mother is concerned because he is complaining of pain in his right ear since last night. She advised she has given him some paracetamol, but he still complains of throbbing. Other than the ear pain he is well in himself. On further investigation, you confirm he is asthmatic and is currently using a clenil modulite and ventolin inhaler. On further exploration you confirm it is likely acute otitis media. What is the most APPROPRIATE treatment plan for this patient at this stage?

☐ A Advise patient to purchase ear calm to alleviate symptoms

☐ B Advise the mother that otitis media is self-limiting, and he should continue with paracetamol. Symptoms can take 3–7 days to resolve and if her son's symptoms persists or worsens to see a GP

☐ C Advise the mother to consider ibuprofen as this can help with the symptoms since otitis media is characterised by inflammation in the middle ear associated with effusion. Ibuprofen can be taken up to three times a day along side the paracetamol so will reduce the throbbing the patient feels between doses

☐ D Refer to A&E

☐ E Refer to GP for antibiotics

184 Mr LN is an 81-year-old man on palliative care treatment. You are working on the elderly care ward in the hospital. The consultant asks that you prescribe something for the patient's dry mouth. Which is the most appropriate treatment for this patient?

☐ A Benzydamine mouth wash

☐ B Chlorhexidine gluconate mouth wash

☐ C Glandosane aerosol spray

☐ D Miconazole oral gel

☐ E NeilMed sinus rinse

185 Mrs KN, a 71-year-old woman with a BMI of 25, has had a flare up of eczema on both of her legs. The dermatologist has requested that she use a moderately potent topical corticosteroid – betnovate RD to help alleviate the flare; she has requested the patient to use it thinly, once a day for two weeks. What is the appropriate amount of betnovate RD to prescribe for this patient?

☐ A 15g
☐ B 30g
☐ C 60g
☐ D 100g
☐ E 200g

186 Most vaccines need to be stored in a refrigerator. What is the usual storage conditions required for most vaccines?

☐ A -1 - 8°C
☐ B 0 - 8°C
☐ C 2 - 8°C
☐ D 6 - 8°C
☐ E 22 - 25°C

187 You receive a prescription in the outpatient pharmacy for emla 5% cream with 2 occlusive dressings for a 10-year-old child. The active ingredient is lidocaine 25mg/1g and prilocaine 25mg/1g. What group of drugs do the active ingredients fall under?

☐ A Anaesthetics
☐ B Antibiotics
☐ C Antiemitics
☐ D Antiretrovirals
☐ E Opiates

188 A 65-year-old man was diagnosed with prostate cancer 2 months ago. He was prescribed zoladex LA (goserelin) to be administered subcutaneously as an alternative to surgical castration. Which one of the following has most likely also been prescribed for this patient as a result of side effects to the goserelin?

☐ A Bicalutamide
☐ B Estradot patches
☐ C Multivitamins
☐ D Orlistat
☐ E Sildenafil

189 Mr JF, a 56-year-old man, visits the community pharmacy to buy some
Nexium tablets. He explains to you that he is experiencing heartburn and
upper abdominal pain which he has not experienced before. A friend
recommended Nexium and it 'works a treat' for Mr JF. Although the
symptoms are becoming worse, he mentions he is feeling quite positive
because the tablets have supressed his appetite and he has now lost weight.
What is the most APPROPRIATE advice for this patient?

☐ A Advise patient to buy Gaviscon in addition to the Nexium to use
when the Nexium wears off

☐ B Book an appointment with the GP, so he can review symptoms and
make a 2-week referral to cancer pathway

☐ C Book an appointment with the GP so he can try some more
common PPI's, e.g. lansoprazole/omeprazole

☐ D Try Gaviscon first as it is the first time, he has had these symptoms

☐ E Try Nexium for 2 weeks, and if no improvement, book an
appointment with the GP

190 Mrs PW, a 46-year-old female patient, has had pain in her right knee
for a few years due to osteoarthritis. This is usually well managed with
paracetamol, ibuprofen 10% gel and regular physiotherapy sessions. She
has an appointment with the Advanced Clinical Practitioner (ACP) to
discuss a flare up of the pain despite using her current pain management.
The ACP would like to discuss possible pain options with you. What
would be the most APPROPRIATE next course of action?

☐ A Change ibuprofen gel to diclofenac gel

☐ B Short course of lowest most effective dose of naproxen

☐ C Short course of tramadol

☐ D Start or increase anaerobic exercise

☐ E More frequent physiotherapy

The next three questions (191-193) are based on the same list of options, but different scenarios. Each option may be used once, more than once or not at all.

Theme – Signposting patients

☐ A Book routine appointment with the GP
☐ B Book same day appointment with the GP
☐ C Prescription needed from walk in centre
☐ D Refer urgently to secondary care specialist
☐ E Self-care advice
☐ F Treat with over the counter product
☐ G Urgent referral to A&E
☐ H None of the above

191 A 27-year-old female patient has some pain in her left eye which is also red and quite sore. On questioning, you find that the pain started since she changed her contact lenses yesterday morning. What should you advise the patient to do?

192 A 43-year-old man presents with a sore throat to the community pharmacy. It is causing slight discomfort when he is eating and drinking. On observation, you notice he has inflamed tonsils but no other symptoms. What is the most APPROPRIATE action to take?

193 A 35-year-old mum of a 5-year-old girl comes into the pharmacy to discuss her concerns. She thinks her daughter is suffering with a dry scalp due to frequent itching. She asks you to review in order to confirm this diagnosis. During the examination, you spot head lice walking across the top of her hair. Which course of action should you take?

194 A father of a 12-month-old baby girl wants to enquire about two outstanding vaccines for his daughter. He does not have many days off work so ideally would like them to be administered on the same day but wants to check this would be safe to do so. The outstanding vaccines are bacillus calmette-guérin (BCG) vaccine and the measles, mumps and rubella (MMR) vaccine. What is the correct advice for this parents' enquiry?

☐ A The vaccines are both live and so MUST be 4 weeks apart

☐ B The vaccines are both live and should either be administered on the same day or 4 weeks apart, but should preferably be administered on different limbs

☐ C The vaccines can be administered on the same day and on the same or different limb

☐ D The vaccines can be administered on the same day, but the BCG must be administered first

☐ E The vaccines can be administered on the same day, but the MMR must be administered first

195 You are a hospital pharmacist working on the orthopaedics ward. A 35-year-old woman is due to have surgery on her left knee following an injury a few months ago. On reviewing her current list of medicines, the anaesthetist decides he is going to continue one of her repeat medications during anaesthesia. Which one of the following is most likely to be continued and for what reason?

☐ A Amitriptyline, due to discontinuation of symptoms

☐ B Long term prednisolone due to the risk of a precipitous fall in blood pressure

☐ C Microgynon due to the risk of getting pregnant

☐ D Ramipril due to the risk of hypertension

☐ E Spironolactone due to the risk of hypokalaemia

196 You are a general practice pharmacist reconciling a letter from an ophthalmology clinic for a patient who has glaucoma. The letter advises to continue latanoprost 50mcg/ml eye drops once a day both eyes for long term but didn't specify what time of the day to instil the drops. Which of the following time frame is latanoprost recommended to be administered?

☐ A Any time of the day

☐ B Bedtime

☐ C Evening

☐ D Lunch time

☐ E Morning

197 You are working in a community pharmacy. A 19-year-old patient has requested to purchase an intranasal topical corticosteroid spray for allergic rhinitis. He has already tried oral antihistamines but they have not been effective. The patient has requested to purchase a particular intranasal topical corticosteroid however the spray he has requested is a prescription-only medication (POM). Which of the following intranasal corticosteroid has the patient likely requested?

☐ A Beconase hayfever relief for adults (beclometasone)
☐ B Nasonex allergy control (mometasone) nasal spray
☐ C Nasacort allergy relief (triamcinolone) nasal spray
☐ D Pirinase hayfever relief (fluticasone) for adults
☐ E Pollenase hayfever relief (beclometasone) for adults

198 An 11-year-old girl has had a flare up of eczema despite using emollients regularly. She has been using a mild topical corticosteroid, but this has not settled the flare up. You have been asked to recommend a moderate potency corticosteroid. Which of the following would be the most appropriate to use?

☐ A Beclometasone dipropionate 0.025%
☐ B Betamethasone valerate 0.025%
☐ C Clobetasol 0.05%
☐ D Diflucortolone valerate 0.1%
☐ E Hydrocortisone butyrate 0.1%

199 A 64-year-old male patient is due to have a vaccine when they are 65 years old. You are a community pharmacist and have been asked to clarify which injection the patient will be likely to receive at this age aside from the annual influenza vaccine. Assuming the patient is up to date with their vaccinations, which of the following vaccines is the patient likely to receive next?

☐ A Herpes-zoster vaccine
☐ B Meningitis B (1st dose)
☐ C Meningitis B (2nd dose)
☐ D Pneumococcal polysaccharide vaccine
☐ E Rotavirus (2nd dose)

200 A 40-year-old patient is due to undergo a complex surgical operation. You are a surgical pharmacist and have been asked by an anaesthetist to recommend an anaesthetic that is long acting and has non-depolarising neuromuscular blocking properties. Which of the following of the following would be the most appropriate to recommend?

☐ A Atracurium besilate
☐ B Mivacurium
☐ C Pancuronium bromide
☐ D Rocuronium bromide
☐ E Vecuronium bromide

201 You are due to have a patient safety meeting with the local GP practice. To attend the meeting you have signed yourself absent as the responsible pharmacist (from the community pharmacy) in the pharmacy record. A pharmacy technician wonders what activities can take place whilst you are away. Which of the following activities cannot take place without the physical presence of a pharmacist?

☐ A Accuracy checking
☐ B Handing out dispensed medicine to the delivery driver
☐ C Processing waste stock medicine (excluding CDs)
☐ D Receiving prescription directly from patients
☐ E Responding to enquiries (about medicine issues)

202 You are working in a community pharmacy. The controlled drug register is almost full, and you have been asked by a trainee pharmacist how long to keep a CD register after it is fully completed. Which of the following time frames would be most appropriate to advise?

☐ A For 1 year from the date of the first entry
☐ B For 2 years from the date of the last entry
☐ C For 3 years from the date of the last entry
☐ D For 5 years from the date of the first entry
☐ E For 5 years from the date of the last entry

203 Which piece of legislation defines the labelling requirements for medicines dispensed in England?

☐ A Human Medicines Regulations (2012)
☐ B Misuse of Drugs Act
☐ C The Medicines Act (1968)
☐ D The Pharmacy Order (2010)
☐ E None of the above

204 What schedule in the Misuse of Drugs Regulations does pregabalin fall into?

☐ A Schedule 1
☐ B Schedule 2
☐ C Schedule 3
☐ D Schedule 4a
☐ E Schedule 5

205 You are a hospital-based pharmacist working on the respiratory ward. You work closely alongside an advanced clinical practitioner who is a paramedic by background. They check if they are able to prescribe unlicensed medication with yourself. Pharmacists, and which other independent prescriber may prescribe unlicensed medicines?

☐ A Nurse/midwife
☐ B Optometrist
☐ C Paramedic
☐ D Podiatrist/chiropodist
☐ E Therapeutic radiographer

206 You are a community pharmacist and you have been assigned the role of training all the dispensing staff on processing prescriptions. Which of the following is NOT a legal requirement on a UK prescription?

☐ A Address of the prescriber
☐ B Age of the patient if under 16 years
☐ C Name of the patient
☐ D Signature of the prescriber
☐ E Written in indelible ink

207 Mrs LR (31-years-old) attends your community pharmacy and advises you that she is on holiday in the area and has forgotten her medicines. Which of the following is NOT a requirement for supplying an emergency supply?

- [ ] A A POM must have been used as a treatment and prescribed by a UK, EEA or Swiss health professional
- [ ] B The maximum quantity for a POM supplied under emergency supply is 30 days
- [ ] C The pharmacist must be confident of the dose prescribed
- [ ] D The pharmacist must interview the patient
- [ ] E The pharmacist must receive payment for the medication supplied

208 Dr PL would like to give his patient enough clobetasone to treat her flare up of psoriasis which is active on her knees, elbows, and arms. It is likely it will need to be used for 2-4 weeks. The cream is available in 30g and 100g tubes. You are based in a prescribing clinic alongside Dr PL. How much should be prescribed?

- [ ] A 60g
- [ ] B 100g
- [ ] C 130g
- [ ] D 160g
- [ ] E 200g

209 Choose the CORRECT statement regarding professional standards. Pharmacy professionals must:

- [ ] A Apply the same high standards when using social media as used in face-to-face interactions
- [ ] B Avoid being open and honest with patients when things go wrong
- [ ] C Hold sufficient indemnity cover for all professional and personal activities they undertake
- [ ] D Not declare potential conflict of interests
- [ ] E Revalidate their registration with the General Pharmaceutical Council every 2 years

210 Roaccutane is being prescribed for Miss JL (19-years-old) due to her severe acne. You receive a prescription for her medication. Which of the following is a correct statement regarding this medication?

☐ A A maximum of 28 days to be supplied on the prescription
☐ B Kidney function should be checked every 3 months
☐ C Miss JL should have signed up for the pregnancy prevention programme
☐ D Roaccutane should not be prescribed by brand name
☐ E The medication should be issued as a whole per course (e.g., 8 weeks course treatment to be issued)

The next five questions (211-215) are based on the same list of options, but different scenarios. Each option may be used once, more than once, or not at all.

Themes: Bloods

☐ A Alfacalcidol capsules
☐ B Colecalciferol capsules
☐ C Ferrous sulphate tablets
☐ D Folic acid tablets
☐ E Hydroxocobalamin IM
☐ F Levothyroxine tablets
☐ G Thiamine tablets
☐ H Vitamin B12 tablets

211 A 25-year-old pregnant female has been advised to take this in her first trimester to prevent the risks of spina bifida.

212 A 51-year-old female has been diagnosed with pernicious anaemia (has confirmed vitamin B12 deficiency).

213 A 28-year-old male patient with low vitamin D levels and has been advised to buy this in the low dose version over the counter due to symptoms of tiredness.

214 A 35-year-old patient who was prescribed this medicine (after checking blood levels) and presented with the following symptoms: weight gain, constipation, puffy face, tiredness, joint pain, irregular menses.

215 A 52-year-old male who has been prescribed this medication due to the risk of Wernicke-Korsakoff.

Additional questions: Mixture of High, Medium and Low

216 You are a practice pharmacist working in a minor ailment's clinic. You have reviewed a 4-year-old male child presenting with a seal like barking cough. Upon chest auscultation you identify the child has stridor. The mother explains the symptoms are worse at night. You note the child has a mild fever and can eat and drink. There is no family history of respiratory diseases. No other members of the family are affected, and they have not travelled abroad recently. Which of the following is the likely diagnosis?

☐ A Common cold
☐ B COVID-19
☐ C Croup
☐ D Cystic fibrosis
☐ E Tuberculosis

217 A mental health nurse has reviewed a 15-year-old female patient. The patient was referred to cognitive behaviour therapy (CBT) for low mood but found it ineffective; she would like to trial an antidepressant. Which of the following antidepressants would be the most appropriate for this patient?

☐ A Amitriptyline
☐ B Fluoxetine
☐ C Moclobemide
☐ D Paroxetine
☐ E Venlafaxine

218 A 10-year-old male child has presented to your community pharmacy with his mother. The child has small, erythematous macules on the scalp, face, trunk, and proximal limbs which are very itchy. The mother believes the child caught it from school as there has been an outbreak of chickenpox. The child is able to eat and drink and is well in himself. You agree the likely diagnosis is chickenpox. The mother asks for advice on how to manage chickenpox. Which of the following advice would be the LEAST appropriate to provide?

- ☐ A Avoid contact with people who are immunocompromised, pregnant women and infants aged 4 weeks or less
- ☐ B Chlorphenamine can be used for treating itch
- ☐ C Ibuprofen can be used to manage pain or fever
- ☐ D Keep away from school until all the vesicles have crusted over
- ☐ E Keep nails short to minimise damage from scratching and secondary bacterial infection from scratching

219 You are working in a community pharmacy and have received a Community Pharmacy Consultation Service (CPCS) referral for a number of patients with suspected conjunctivitis. You diagnose each patient with bacterial conjunctivitis. Before you sell the medication, you review if over-the-counter chloramphenicol would be suitable for them. Which of the following patients would it be most appropriate to sell chloramphenicol?

- ☐ A A 20-year-old patient presenting with a red eye
- ☐ B A 23-year-old patient who is 20 weeks pregnant
- ☐ C A 34-year-old patient who wears contact lens
- ☐ D A 45-year-old patient with severe pain within the affected eye
- ☐ E A 56-year-old patient with a history of glaucoma

220 You are a community pharmacist reviewing outstanding New Medicine Service consultations. You have identified a patient that is not eligible for the service as per the service specification. Which of the following patient would not be eligible for the service?

- ☐ A A patient who has started a new diabetes (type 1) medication
- ☐ B A patient who has started a new epilepsy medication

☐ C A patient who has started a new hypercholesterolaemia medication
☐ D A patient who has started a new hypertension medication
☐ E A patient who has started a new Parkinson's disease medication

221 A trainee pharmacist is creating a list of medications that can be sold as General Sale List (GSL) medicine to help him prepare for the GPhC registration exam. Which of the following products should be included in the list?

☐ A Chloramphenicol 1% (optrex) eye ointment
☐ B Fexofenadine 120mg (allevia) tablets
☐ C Lidocaine 1% (anbesol) oral teething gel
☐ D Orlistat 60 mg (alli) capsule
☐ E Tamsulosin 0.4mg (flomax relief) modified-release capsule

222 A 73-years-old male is living in a care home. The carer looking after him notices he has a stockpile of medication. His topiramate tablet states 'use by Jan 2025' printed on the box. What is the last day this medication can be taken?

☐ A 31st Dec 2024
☐ B 1st Jan 2025
☐ C 15th Jan 2025
☐ D 31st Jan 2025
☐ E 1st Feb 2025

The next four questions (223-226) are based on the same list of options, but different scenarios. Each option may be used once, more than once or not at all.

Which out of the following options is the MOST likely diagnosis for each question?

☐ A Chickenpox
☐ B Colic
☐ C Cow's milk allergy
☐ D Croup
☐ E IBS

☐ F Measles
☐ G Meningitis
☐ H Scarlet fever

223 An 11-week-old baby boy has been crying inconsolably for the last 3-4 weeks for 4-5 hours every day. He is otherwise well fed and healthy.

224 A 2-year-old child has cough and cold symptoms and looks quite unwell. On observation, you find he has a fever and seems to be quite agitated. His mum describes his cough as a very loud barking cough and mentions that he has not been as active as he usually is.

225 A 9-year-old girl has come up with a very itchy rash which started as small red lumps and has now turned into blisters. Her mum mentions that some of the blisters have burst and crusted over, and that there are also some in the mouth. She also describes that she had been feeling unwell and had a fever a couple of days before the rash came up.

226 A 1-year-old baby has a rash that the mum explains does not blanch under pressure when she has tried the glass test. The baby is also more drowsy than usual, has a high temperature and is refusing feeds.

227 A 22-year-old has come to her local pharmacy to seek some advice about her recent symptoms. She initially wondered if these may be related to a cold. Her symptoms started in May, and it is currently July. She is sneezing excessively; has itchy, watery eyes and cannot seem to focus on any of her daily tasks, particularly her studies. Which of the following OTC product would be the most appropriate option to recommend?

☐ A Beconase nasal spray
☐ B Cetirizine tablets
☐ C Loratadine tablets
☐ D Olopatadine eye drops
☐ E Sodium cromoglicate

228 A 58-year-old patient visits your community pharmacy seeking advice regarding his constipation. Upon reviewing, you note he is awaiting a

total knee replacement (TKR) on his left knee. He has been prescribed Zomorph 10mg capsules BD recently. Which of the following laxatives would you recommend that this patient buys OTC to manage his symptoms?

☐ A Bisacodyl
☐ B Docusate and lactulose
☐ C Fybogel sachets
☐ D Lactulose and senna
☐ E Naloxegol

229 A parent of a 1-year-old toddler enters the pharmacy to seek advice on buying multivitamin drops for her baby. She does not mind which flavour but mentions that the baby does have a nut allergy. Which of the following would be safe to recommend?

☐ A Abidec drops
☐ B Dalivit drops
☐ C HalibOrange liquid
☐ D Pro D3 drops
☐ E Wellbaby liquid

230 MK is a 47-year-old builder who works 8-12 hours per day. He visits the community pharmacy and informs you that he does not have time to make a GP appointment and would like to buy an OTC product to help with his symptoms. He has excessive itching in between his toes and the skin around those areas is red, flaky, and quite sore; particularly between the fourth and fifth webspace. Which of the following products SHOULD be recommended?

☐ A Calamine lotion
☐ B Flexitol balm
☐ C Fluconazole capsule
☐ D Hydrocortisone cream
☐ E Terbinafine cream

231 A 76-year-old woman (Mrs PW) presents to the community pharmacy to purchase an item to treat her sore mouth. On observation you notice white plaques and confirm that she has oral thrush. She is a regular patient and is on the following list of medication:

- Clenil modulite 100mcg inhaler
- Salbutamol 100mcg evohaler
- Warfarin 1mg tablets
- Warfarin 3mg tablets

Mrs PW confirms that she has had treatment supplied OTC in the past for a sore mouth. Which of the following is the most appropriate action to take?

- ☐ A Advise her to wait 7-10 days as the thrush may go away on its own
- ☐ B Recommend that she buys chlorhexidine mouth wash
- ☐ C Recommend that she buys miconazole oral gel
- ☐ D Recommend that she buys nystatin oral suspension
- ☐ E Refer to GP surgery to get a prescription for nystatin oral suspension

232 Ms FC, a 44-year-old patient, visits the community pharmacy seeking your advice. She has travelled from outside of the city and is staying with her sister. She was due to travel back home yesterday and thought she had enough of her repeat medicines however due to personal circumstances, her travel plans have been delayed and she will now be out of her regular medication tomorrow. She requests an emergency supply. Her regular repeat medication is:

- Ramipril 5mg capsules
- Metformin 1g MR tablets

Which of the following is a condition that applies when an emergency supply is requested by a patient?

- ☐ A A prescription has to be provided to the pharmacy within 72 hours
- ☐ B The patient may not have had the medication previously
- ☐ C The prescription only medicine can be a schedule 2 controlled drug

☐ D You are satisfied that there is an immediate need for the emergency supply

☐ E You should not interview the patient if their relative is present

233 You are the responsible pharmacist at the community pharmacy. You receive a prescription from the local surgery for a known patient. The prescription is for MST continus 30mg tablets. The pharmacy technician whilst labelling notices that it may not be legally accurate to dispense but wants to double check with yourself. Which of the following CAN be amended by pharmacists on a controlled drug prescription?

☐ A Add 'for dental treatment only' if missing on a dental prescription

☐ B Add quantity in words or figures if missing in one or the other but not both

☐ C The date on the prescription if over 28 days but you have spoken to the prescriber, and they still intend to prescribe it

☐ D The dose if it just says 'as directed'

☐ E The strength of the medication if you do not have the prescribed one in stock

234 Mr GH (age 44 years) is under the local addiction services and is prescribed methadone solution on an FP10MDA prescription which he brings to your pharmacy. Mr GH is usually supervised on a daily basis but wonders what will happen on the upcoming bank holiday. Which of the following is the MOST APPROPRIATE answer?

☐ A A new prescription is needed from the addiction services team to cover the bank holiday

☐ B Mr Hughes may need to contact the out of hours team on the day the pharmacy is closed

☐ C Mr Hughes must go back to the addiction services for them to provide the methadone on the day the Pharmacy is closed

☐ D The pharmacist can hand out the methadone supply on a day prior the date the Pharmacy is closed as long as the prescription contains the specific home office wording

☐ E There are no specific requirements needed and the methadone supply can be handed out a day prior to the day the pharmacy is closed

235 Mrs EB (age 62 years) is a regular patient at the pharmacy you work in and over the years, you have managed to build a rapport with her as she regularly brings her repeat prescriptions. You actioned a medication review 2 months ago and identified that she had been trying to lose weight due to an overweight BMI (27 kg/m2). You notice on today's prescription that Mrs EB has been prescribed a new medicine – pioglitazone. After discussing, you confirm that she has recently been diagnosed with type two diabetes. Which of the following action should you take?

☐ A Check the prescription for clinical and dispensing accuracy as you assume there must be a contraindication to metformin which is first line

☐ B Discuss with the reception team at the surgery to see if there are any notes around prescribing choice

☐ C Do not challenge the prescriber as they have the patients' full notes and will have made an informed decision

☐ D Refer Mrs EB to the prescriber

☐ E Set up a telephone consultation with the prescriber to discuss rationale behind the prescribing choice

236 Mrs SK (33-years-old) visits your community pharmacy to buy a thermometer to measure her infants temperature. She informs you her infant is 3 weeks old and is concerned regarding a raised temperature. In infants under the age of 4 weeks, what is the most appropriate way to measure the infant's body temperature?

☐ A Forehead

☐ B In the axilla

☐ C Oral

☐ D Rectal

☐ E None of the above

237 Miss LA, a 6-year-old child, comes into the community pharmacy with her mother. Her mother is concerned with a rash that has started on her stomach. On observation you notice that there are small fluid filled red lumps and that they seem to be spreading on to her legs and forming on her hands. Miss LA advises they are itchy. Her Mother informs you that

other than the rash and the itchiness she is well in herself, although she has recently recovered from a cold. Based on the patient's symptoms what is the likely diagnosis for this patient?

☐ A Chickenpox
☐ B Impetigo
☐ C Measles
☐ D Molluscum contagiosum
☐ E Shingles

238 Miss GC, a 10-year-old girl, has been diagnosed by the doctor as having the 'kissing disease.' The patient complains of fatigue and sore throat, and on examination the doctor sees that the patients lymph nodes are swollen. Based on the patient's symptoms what is the likely diagnosis for this patient?

☐ A Erythema infectiosum
☐ B German measles
☐ C Glandular fever (infectious mononucleosis)
☐ D Meningitis
☐ E Mumps

239 Baby LR, a 6-month-old baby girl, comes into the GP surgery with her father. You are a prescribing pharmacist managing acutely unwell patients. You have been asked to review baby LR. The father is concerned as she has developed a rash on her bum which he shows you. On examination you note a bright red rash. It is sore and has some well defined papular lesions. You undertake a full body examination and also note some lesions are present on her hands. Baby LR is in a lot of discomfort and cries mainly when nappies are changed. What is the most appropriate treatment option for this patient?

☐ A Clotrimazole 1% cream
☐ B Metanium
☐ C Sudocream
☐ D Vaseline
☐ E No treatment is required as it is a self-limiting condition

240 You are a community pharmacist reviewing a prescription for a 3-month-old baby (Baby ZN). The doctor has prescribed ibuprofen 100mg/5ml oral solution - 100mg three times a day. Which of the following statements is CORRECT?

    □ A Dose is incorrect, it should be 50mg three times a day for a 3-month year old

    □ B Dose is incorrect, it should be 200mg three times a day for a 3-month year old

    □ C Ibuprofen 100mg/5ml oral solution does not exist

    □ D Ibuprofen is not indicated in a patient at 3 months

    □ E There is nothing wrong with this prescription

241 You are a hospital pharmacist working on a paediatrics ward. The trainee pharmacist is shadowing you whilst you undertake your clinical reviews. She asks you about fevers in children. You advise her that fever in children can be considered serious. In which case should referral to the emergency services NOT be considered?

    □ A Febrile convulsions

    □ B Fever accompanied with no other symptoms

    □ C Fever for 3 days

    □ D Signs of dehydration

    □ E Stiff neck

242 Miss FR, a 43-year-old woman, presents to the community pharmacy with a bright red segment in the left eye only. She informs you that it isn't painful and other than having a bit of a cough she is otherwise well in herself. She is concerned because it looks bad in appearance. Based on the patients' symptoms what is the most likely diagnosis?

    □ A Keratitis

    □ B Scelritis

    □ C Subconjunctival haemorrhage

    □ D Uveitis

    □ E Viral conjunctivitis

243 Mr PL, a 55-year-old man, presents to the community pharmacy with a small black dot on the heel of his foot, he describes it as being extremely painful especially when he is walking. You ask whether he takes any other medication, and he informs you that he is currently taking:

- Metformin 500mg tablets – ONE twice a day
- Co-codamol 8/500mg tablets – ONE or TWO to be taken up to four times a day
- Lansoprazole 30mg capsules – ONE daily

What is the most appropriate treatment plan for this patient?

☐ **A** Bazuka extra strength
☐ **B** Duofilm
☐ **C** Refer to GP
☐ **D** Salactol
☐ **E** Silver nitrate

244 Miss EG, a 21-year-old woman, comes into the pharmacy with her 2-year-old son. She is concerned with little red marks that are appearing on the webs of his fingers and the sides of his hand. He seems to be scratching them profusely. She mentioned that he was playing with her niece the other day who had the similar redness in between her fingers and was wondering whether it was anything that was contagious. You examine the patient and you diagnose him with scabies. Which of the following statements is INCORRECT with regards to scabies and the treatment of scabies?

☐ **A** Clothes towels and bed linen should be machine washed at (50 degrees celsius or above) at the time of first application to prevent reinfestation and transmitting to others.
☐ **B** Itching can persist for 2 – 3 weeks after treatment.
☐ **C** It is important that all people in the same household and in close contact with the affected are treated at the same time to prevent reinfection, even though they may be asymptomatic.
☐ **D** Permethrin is the first line of choice and a whole tube should be used on everyone in the household as a single application. Some adults may need more than one tube to cover their body.
☐ **E** Treatment should not be applied after a hot bath because this increases systemic absorption and removes the drug from the treatment site.

245 Mebendazole is available over the counter for the treatment of threadworms. Which medication decreases mebendazole plasma levels resulting in the potential need for an increased dose of mebendazole?

☐ A Amlodipine
☐ B Carbamazepine
☐ C Digoxin
☐ D Gliclazide
☐ E Sodium valproate

246 A patient visits the community pharmacy requesting diphenhydramine (Nytol) as a sleep aid. Which patient from the list below can you supply the medication to?

☐ A Miss AM, an 11-year-old girl, who struggles to sleep at night because of the amount of pressure she feels she is under. Her mother comes in requesting some Nytol to help her to get some sleep as she is becoming quite distressed due to the lack of sleep.

☐ B Miss HM, a 25-year-old woman, who works as an air hostess has recently come off night flights and has been put on day flights, which she is struggling with as she can't sleep at night. She is requesting Nytol for a short term to help with her altered sleep pattern.

☐ C Mr AA, a 21-year-old man who takes fluoxetine, advises he struggles to sleep at night for months on end as he is in a lot of pain and would like to try Nytol to see if that can help him to sleep.

☐ D Mr AS, a 62-year-old man, who has been unable to sleep since the passing of his wife two months ago. He advises he is quite distressed and is therefore unable to sleep and would like some Nytol to help him sleep at night.

☐ E Mrs PM, a 78-year-old woman, who struggles to sleep at night due to the sounds she can hear. She advises she is a light sleeper and has struggled to sleep for years. She saw on TV that Nytol could help with sleep and would like to try to see if it will help.

247 Miss TB, a 33-year-old woman, visits the community pharmacy complaining of itchiness in her vaginal area which is associated with a white discharge. She is wondering what the most appropriate treatment is. She is not pregnant and is currently taking the progesterone only pill. Which medication would NOT be suitable for this patient?

☐ A Canesten duo
☐ B Clotrimazole 2% cream
☐ C Clotrimazole 500mg pessary
☐ D Fluconazole 150mg oral capsule
☐ E Ketoconazole 2% cream

248 Ms JH, a 58-year-old woman, comes into the pharmacy complaining of thrush-like symptoms She informs you that she used to 'get it in her younger years but it has been years since she last had it'. Ms JH is not sexually active and washes her vaginal area with water only; she wears loosely fitted clothing and hasn't changed her washing powder. You ask her about her recent medication intake. Which medication from the list below is most likely to have contributed to the thrush?

☐ A Bisoprolol
☐ B Co-amoxiclav
☐ C Dihydrocodeine
☐ D Naproxen
☐ E Ramipril

249 Mrs TH, a 44-year-old woman, comes into the community pharmacy presenting with pain in her stomach. On examination you note it is in her upper abdomen. The pain is described as a 'burning sensation' that seems to get worse after eating. She informs you that 'it keeps her up at night' and is requesting medication for this. On further exploration you are satisfied that the patient is suffering from gastritis. Which of the following medication is a POM medication?

☐ A Esomeprazole
☐ B Gaviscon
☐ C Rabeprazole
☐ D Ranitidine
☐ E Rennies

250 Mr IP, a 41-year-old man, presents to the pharmacy with a red, dry, thick, scaling lesion of patches on his right elbow. It looks quite irritated, as though he has been itching it. Mr IP is not in any pain and is not aware of any insect bites. What is the most likely diagnosis for this patient?

☐ A Dermatitis
☐ B Eczema
☐ C Plaque psoriasis
☐ D Ringworm
☐ E Scabies

251 Mrs KJ, a 59-year-old woman, presents to the community pharmacy with pain in her back. Mrs KJ thinks it started after picking up something heavy. She is currently in the process of moving house and has been heavy lifting. You ask her whether she is on any other regular medication, and she informs you that she currently takes:

- Ramipril 10mg capsules
- QVAR 100mcg inhaler
- Ventolin 100mcg evohaler

She informs you she has not tried anything for the pain yet. What is the most appropriate treatment plan for this patient?

☐ A Aspirin 300mg PO PRN
☐ B Ibuprofen 5% topical up to QDS PRN
☐ C Ibuprofen 400mg PO up to TDS PRN
☐ D Paracetamol PO 1g QDS
☐ E Naproxen 250mg PO BD PRN

252 Mr BK, a 40-year-old man, presents to the community pharmacy with hay fever symptoms. His eyes are itching, he has a runny nose and is sneezing frequently. He has requested an antihistamine but advises that he is a bus driver and works during the day. Which is the most appropriate antihistamine for this patient?

☐ A Chlorphenamine

☐ B Cinnarizine
☐ C Hydroxyzine
☐ D Loratadine
☐ E Promethazine

253 Miss KK, a 38-year-old woman, presents to the community pharmacy with a strong headache. She describes this as being all over the front of her head and it feels as though it is quite tight as though something is pressing down on it. She has a regular partner, 2 children and a highly stressful financial job. Based on the description of her symptoms, what is her likely diagnosis from the list below?

☐ A Cluster headache
☐ B Glaucoma
☐ C Sinusitis
☐ D Subarachnoid haemorrhage
☐ E Tension

254 Mr LS, a 40-year-old patient, comes into your community pharmacy requesting something for his cough. It is a productive cough that he has had for three days and he is requesting a medication that will help lift it off his chest. He is not currently taking any medication and doesn't smoke. He has not tried anything but advises that his wife is a nurse and she told him to increase his fluid intake which he has been doing. Which is the more appropriate treatment for this patient?

☐ A Dextromethorphan
☐ B Glycerine, honey and lemon
☐ C Guafanesin
☐ D Pholcodine
☐ E Referral to GP

255 Miss SH, a 28-year-old patient, comes into your community pharmacy requesting Solpadeine Max tablets. You note she presented a few days earlier requesting the same medication. She advises you that it is for her back pain that she has had for a while now and she doesn't want to get it on prescription because the prescription is more expensive and she pays

for her medication. What statement is CORRECT with regards to the management of this patient?

- [ ] A Advise patient to purchase low strength co-codamol 8/500mg tablets as they are cheaper
- [ ] B Refer patient to A&E as the pain may be uncontrolled
- [ ] C Refer patient to GP as codeine containing products are restricted to a short-term (3 days) treatment of acute pain
- [ ] D Refer to GP as Solpadeine Max is a prescription only medication
- [ ] E Sell Miss SH the Solpadeine as she is taking it for her back and therefore this is likely chronic so the patient is in need of this.

256 Mrs JB, a 65-year-old woman, has been given a prescription by her neurology specialist for:

- Gabapentin 300mg capsules – take ONE three times a day (168)

Mrs JB presents to the community pharmacy with this prescription. Which of the following statements is CORRECT?

- [ ] A Gabapentin dose is incorrect
- [ ] B Gabapentin is not available as 300mg
- [ ] C Gabapentin is not available as capsules
- [ ] D The number of gabapentin capsules to be dispensed is not allowed
- [ ] E There is nothing wrong with this prescription

257 Mrs GF (63 years) presents with a prescription for Zomorph capsules 10mg BD. You are the responsible pharmacist on site. You are validating the prescription. How long is a controlled drug prescription valid for?

- [ ] A 28 days
- [ ] B 3 months
- [ ] C 6 months
- [ ] D 12 months
- [ ] E It does not have an expiry date

258 Which of the following is good practice in the legal aspects of prescription writing?

- ☐ **A** Address of the prescriber and indication of the type of prescriber
- ☐ **B** A valid date
- ☐ **C** Name of patient
- ☐ **D** The weight of the patient where it has been used to determine dose
- ☐ **E** Written or printed legibly in indelible ink

259 Which schedule of controlled drugs requires a register?

- ☐ **A** Schedule 1
- ☐ **B** Schedule 2
- ☐ **C** Schedule 3
- ☐ **D** Schedule 4
- ☐ **E** Schedule 5

260 Which of the following is a legal requirement for the responsible pharmacist?

- ☐ **A** Displaying a notice that gives the details of who the responsible pharmacist is
- ☐ **B** Pharmacy procedures to be recorded in writing, electronic forms are not acceptable
- ☐ **C** The responsible pharmacist is responsible for all of the pharmacy staff and must ensure their wellbeing and care
- ☐ **D** The responsible pharmacist must be on the premises at all times, absences are in breach of the law
- ☐ **E** The responsible pharmacist must put aside their personal views and should participate in all aspects of care including the administration of the morning after pill

261 Pharmacy professionals must speak up when they have concerns or when things go wrong. This is a professional standard. What is a CORRECT statement regarding this professional standard?

- ☐ **A** Challenge poor practice and behaviors when it only concerns you
- ☐ **B** Do not promote and encourage a culture of learning and improvement
- ☐ **C** Promptly tell employers regarding concerns but relevant authorities need not be included

☐ D Reflect on feedback or concerns, taking action as appropriate and thinking about what can be done to prevent the same thing from happening again

☐ E Reprimand those who raise a concern and provide feedback

262 Master ZM (9 months) presents to the community pharmacy with a widespread itchy rash. Mum informs you it presented as a faint red spot initially and over the past 2 days it has spread on the stomach, face, back and legs. Master ZM is struggling to sleep at night due to the itching. What is the most appropriate plan of action?

☐ A Refer to A&E

☐ B Refer to GP

☐ C Supply chlorphenamine liquid (Piriton)

☐ D Supply loratadine liquid

☐ E Supply paracetamol liquid

263 You are a community pharmacist working at your local pharmacy. Mrs BP presents with a query about her 7-year-old daughter (MS). She has been complaining about an itchy bottom and mum has noticed thread like residue on the bedsheets today. From the review, you decide to act as this is looking like a likely diagnosis of threadworms. Which of the following is a correct statement regarding the sale of mebendazole?

☐ A All cases of threadworms should be referred to a GP

☐ B Do not supply to children under the age of 1 years

☐ C Do not supply to family members

☐ D Take a further dose after 2 weeks if reinfection is suspected

☐ E Take one tablet once a day for 2 weeks

264 Mrs FV (23 years) presents to the community pharmacy requesting the morning after pill. You are the responsible pharmacist and unprotected sexual intercourse took place 24 hours ago. Mrs FV takes nil regular medication and is not currently prescribed any regular medication. She has nil allergies. Her BMI is 24.5m2. Which of the following is a CORRECT statement?

- [ ] **A** If ellaOne is supplied, then you must inform the patient it will only work if regular contraceptive medication is co-prescribed
- [ ] **B** If ellaOne is supplied, then you must inform the patient to continue with barrier methods until the next period
- [ ] **C** If Levonelle is supplied, then you must inform the patient it will only work if regular contraceptive medication is co-prescribed
- [ ] **D** If Levonelle is supplied, then you must inform the patient to continue with barrier methods until the next period
- [ ] **E** This patient requires a GP referral as she has no past history of contraceptive medication

265 Mr KS brings his baby girl (6-weeks-old) to your practice clinic. He is concerned as he has noticed she is not settled during or after breastfeeds and cries constantly. They have tried Infacol drops, and this has made no difference. There is no history of blood in her vomit or stools. Which statement is FALSE?

- [ ] **A** A trial without treatment should occur every 2 weeks
- [ ] **B** Breast-fed infants should be referred for a breastfeeding assessment by a professional with appropriate training and expertise
- [ ] **C** Gaviscon Infant can be trialled for 1-2 weeks
- [ ] **D** Omeprazole may be trialled first-line
- [ ] **E** Symptoms of GORD are common in infants and resolve without treatment before the child is 1 year old

266 Miss TF is a 6-year-old with asthma. She has had a salbutamol inhaler since she was 3 years old. On routine review, you notice that she has had a salbutamol inhaler every month for the last 6 months. Which statement is TRUE?

- [ ] **A** FeNO testing should occur routinely to monitor asthma control
- [ ] **B** Inhaled corticosteroids should be prescribed generically for cost-saving purposes
- [ ] **C** Inhaler technique should only be checked at annual review
- [ ] **D** Parents should be the primary source of information to assess asthma symptoms in children
- [ ] **E** The most appropriate add-on therapy is inhaled beclomethasone 100mg twice daily

267 Mr LD, a 32-year-old man with no clinical history to note, attends your pharmacy asking for advice about irritable bowel syndrome. He has recently been diagnosed by his GP following tests. His main symptoms are bloating, urgency, and flatulence. Mr LD is a truck driver and when on the road, has little opportunity to access fresh fruit and vegetables and can be sat for hours at a time. Which statement is FALSE?

- ☐ A Medication may be considered if dietary and lifestyle optimisation has not helped
- ☐ B Peppermint oil is an irritant to the mouth and oesophagus; capsules should not be opened and taken orally
- ☐ C Rectal bleeding not associated with haemorrhoids should be investigated
- ☐ D Stress is a common trigger of IBS
- ☐ E You should advise Mr LD to resign from his job to optimise his health

The next five questions (268-272) are based on the same list of options, but different scenarios. Each option may be used once, more than once, or not at all.

Themes: Ear

- ☐ A Ear wax
- ☐ B Otitis externa
- ☐ C Otitis media
- ☐ D Rhinitis
- ☐ E Sinusitis
- ☐ F Tinnitus
- ☐ G Upper respiratory tract infection
- ☐ H Vertigo

268 A 53-year-old patient presents to the community pharmacy with a constant humming and whistling noise in his right ear. He is struggling to sleep at night due to this.

269 A 28-year-old patient presents to the community pharmacy feeling a 'fullness' sensation in both ears. They feel blocked and she has also developed some earache.

270 A 3-year-old patient presents to your clinic at the GP surgery. Mum informs you he has been tugging his ear and has developed a fever. He has been crying frequently and become quite restless. On examination his tympanic membrane is red with moderate bulging. Discharge in the auditory canal is also present.

271 A 42-year-old woman presents to the community pharmacy. She had a cold two weeks ago but some of her symptoms continue to persist. She has a frontal headache and feels as if her nose is blocked. She can feel the pressure on her face.

272 A 25-year-old female patient who presents to the community pharmacy. She is a regular swimmer and thinks she has 'swimmer's ear'. Her symptoms are an itchy and painful right ear. Her pinna is quite tender and the ear canal looks red.

Themes: Constipation

The next five questions (273-277) are based on the same list of options, but different scenarios. Each option may be used once, more than once, or not at all.

- ☐ A Bisacodyl suppository
- ☐ B Docusate capsules
- ☐ C Fleet ready to use enema
- ☐ D Fybogel sachets
- ☐ E Lactulose liquid
- ☐ F Movicol paediatric sachets
- ☐ G Senna tablets
- ☐ H Sodium picosulfate liquid

273 Master AZ (7-years-old) presents to the GP surgery with constipation. He has not had any bowel movement for 10 days. Mum has not trialled anything. Master AZ is well in himself and has no other symptoms.

274 Mrs SN (29 years) is 29 weeks pregnant. This is her second pregnancy. Her first pregnancy was a term baby delivered via normal delivery. She is constipated and would like to purchase something over the counter to manage her symptoms.

275 Miss SG (35 years) presents to the GP surgery with persistent constipation. She is requesting something quick acting (within the hour). Miss SG has nil medical history and is 34 weeks pregnant.

276 Mrs SV (42 years) is being prepared for an elective endoscopy. The consultant has requested her bowels to be evacuated prior to the procedure.

277 Mrs BS (72 years) is prescribed medication for his constipation. This is his first prescription being processed by the community pharmacy. You advise him that this medication needs to be carefully swallowed with water and avoid taking before going to bed. It can take a few days for the full effect and adequate fluid must be taken at each dose.

Themes: Childhood conditions

The next five questions (278-282) are based on the same list of options, but different scenarios. Each option may be used once, more than once, or not at all. For each of the following childhood conditions presenting in general practice, choose the most appropriate treatment:

- ☐ A Admit to hospital
- ☐ B Dexamethasone PO for 10 days
- ☐ C Dexamethasone PO stat
- ☐ D Nebulised budesonide 2mg, repeated every 12 hours until clinical improvement
- ☐ E No treatment required
- ☐ F Prescribe antibiotics as per local guidance
- ☐ G Prescribe antifungals as per local guidance
- ☐ H Simple analgesia

278 Hand, foot and mouth disease management

279 Mild croup in a child of average weight

280 Query bacterial meningitis

281 Acute otitis media with no systemic complications

282 A 1-year-old presenting with threadworms

283 Miss LR, who is 13-years-old, has an egg allergy which triggers an anaphylactic reaction. Miss LR has a growth development delay which means that she has not gone through puberty yet. She weighs 33kg. What should be prescribed for her to use in anaphylactic emergency?

☐ **A** Adrenaline 1mg/ml (1 in 1000) injection 150mcg
☐ **B** Adrenaline 1mg/ml (1 in 1000) injection 300mcg
☐ **C** Adrenaline IM auto-injector 500mcg
☐ **D** Adrenaline IM auto-injector 0.15mg
☐ **E** Adrenaline IM auto-injector 0.3mg

284 Mrs LX is 81-years-old, weighs 42kg and is 158cm tall. She has recently seen her GP complaining of a chesty cough, increased wheezing and a tight chest. She has a PMH of COPD and is under the SALT team due to a reduced ability to swallow following a stroke a few years ago. The GP has diagnosed an acute exacerbation of her COPD and has asked your advice on the oral corticosteroid they should prescribe. Which is the most appropriate choice?

☐ **A** Prednisolone soluble 5mg tablets, 6 tablets daily for 7 days
☐ **B** Prednisolone soluble 5mg tablets, 8 tablets daily for 5 days
☐ **C** Prednisolone soluble 5mg tablets, 42mg daily reducing by 6mg each week then stop
☐ **D** Prednisolone soluble 5mg tablets, 84mg daily for 3 days
☐ **E** Rednisolone gastro-resistant 5mg tablets, 6 tablets daily for 7 days

285 Phyllocontin has been discontinued. Your patient is currently taking 225mg bd. What dose of uniphyllin continus should you prescribe? You have access to the following bulletin: https://www.ncl-mon.nhs.uk/wp-content/uploads/Guidelines/3_Aminophylline.pdf

☐ **A** 200mg bd
☐ **B** 300mg bd

☐ C 400mg bd
☐ D 400mg od
☐ E Check levels and dose according to plasma-theophylline concentration

286 Mrs FB, age 38 years, visits your community pharmacy to buy over the counter (OTC) medication for her 2-year-old son who has developed chickenpox due to a recent outbreak at nursery. Which of the following is a CORRECT statement regarding the OTC supply of pain relief in chickenpox medication?

☐ A Do not supply ibuprofen
☐ B Do not supply paracetamol
☐ C Refer to GP due to no license
☐ D Supply ibuprofen only
☐ E Supply paracetamol only

287 Which of the following is classified as an ANTIMUSCARINIC side effect of amitriptyline?

☐ A Diarrhoea
☐ B Dizziness
☐ C Excessive saliva secretion
☐ D Tachycardia
☐ E Weight loss

288 Mr SC (52 years) presents to your prescribing clinic in primary care with alarming features. He has dyspepsia, unintentional weight loss and abdominal pain. He noticed the symptoms three weeks ago. You fast track him to the gastroenterology team for further investigations. Mr SC is advised two weeks later by the gastroenterologist specialist that he has gastric cancer. Which of the following medication may mask symptoms of gastric cancer?

☐ A Fybogel sachets
☐ B Ibuprofen
☐ C Naproxen

☐ D Pantoprazole

☐ E Piroxicam

289 You are a prescribing pharmacist working within primary care. You manage a case load of patients. Mrs SQ, age 28 years, visits your clinic. She informs you that she is in her third trimester and continues to suffer with reflux symptoms. This is her second pregnancy and she experienced similar symptoms during the first pregnancy. She has tried changing her dietary lifestyle and sleeping posture. She has also been taking peptic liquid but is not finding this effective. She has no known drug allergies and nil medical history. What is the most appropriate next step?

☐ A Continue Peptac liquid and add Gaviscon liquid

☐ B Continue Peptac liquid due to high risk in third trimester

☐ C Refer to midwife due to high risk

☐ D Trial low dose famotidine

☐ E Trial low dose omeprazole

290 Mr MN (84 years) is admitted into hospital with a fall and long lie. You are the hospital pharmacist working on the elderly admissions ward. You review his bloods, medication on admission and past medical history. Which one of the following medications may have contributed to his hypomagnesaemia which was the reason for the fall?

☐ A Atorvastatin

☐ B Codeine

☐ C Lansoprazole

☐ D Mirabegron

☐ E Rivaroxaban

291 Miss CP (29 years) visits the sexual health clinic for contraceptive management and advice. She has a regular partner and no drug allergies/intolerance. She has a family history of VTE and is known for poor compliance of her regular medication. She already has 2 children (age 2 years and 9 months) and is not planning any further pregnancies in the next few years. Which of the following would be the most appropriate contraceptive medication in her case?

- ☐ A Copper intrauterine device
- ☐ B Desogestrel PO OD
- ☐ C Elleste solo MX patches applied twice weekly
- ☐ D Femodene PO PO
- ☐ E Osetrogel cream applied daily

292 Mrs PS (82 years) is having swallowing difficulties. The GP has asked to switch her medication of levothyroxine 125mcg daily to liquid form. What dose of levothyroxine 100mcg/5ml liquid should be taken?

- ☐ A 5.15ml daily
- ☐ B 5.25ml daily
- ☐ C 6ml daily
- ☐ D 6.15ml daily
- ☐ E 6.25ml daily

293 Which of the following drugs can considerably reduce the emergency hormonal contraceptive effect?

- ☐ A Carbamazepine
- ☐ B Phenobarbitol
- ☐ C Topiramate
- ☐ D All of the above
- ☐ E None of the above

294 Mrs SF (34 years) presents to the prescribing clinic with right sided breast pain. Upon examination, her right breast is red, swollen and hard. She has a fever (38.3) and is struggling to sleep. The symptoms have been ongoing for one week now. She has noticed some discharge from her nipples. She has nil allergies and nil past medical history. She is not pregnant or breastfeeding. What is the most appropriate management plan?

- ☐ A Fastrack to cancer specialist for two week review due to breast cancer risk
- ☐ B Prescribe NSAID
- ☐ C Prescribe NSAID and antibiotics
- ☐ D Refer to A&E
- ☐ E Safetynet patient and advise no intervention needed

295 Mrs BW (24 years) is currently breastfeeding her 3-month-old baby. This is her first child and Mrs BW has been struggling with the challenges of motherhood. Prior to delivery, Mrs BW was taking antidepressants which worked well for her depression however she stopped these during pregnancy. Mrs BW visits you at your clinic seeking advice as to which antidepressant she can start to take. Mrs BW was previously taking sertraline. Which of the following is the most appropriate recommendation?

☐ **A** Can restart sertraline
☐ **B** To start amitriptyline
☐ **C** To start nortriptyline
☐ **D** To start paroxetine
☐ **E** To start selegiline

296 Mr LS, a 62-year-old man, has been booked in to see the GP because his HbA1c concentration was 62mmol/mol. He is currently on metformin 1g twice a day. The GP advises that he wants to add in another antidiabetic agent but is concerned with severe hypoglycaemia. Which drug is most commonly associated with severe hypoglycaemia?

☐ **A** Canagliflozin
☐ **B** Gliclazide
☐ **C** Liraglutide
☐ **D** Pioglitazone
☐ **E** Sitagliptin

297 Mrs LA, a 52-year-old woman, has been started on ferrous sulfate 200mg BD. How much iron does each dose contain?

☐ **A** 35mg
☐ **B** 45mg
☐ **C** 65mg
☐ **D** 90mg
☐ **E** 130mg

298 Mr PK, a 60-year-old man, has been started on spironolactone for oedema. You are a heart failure management pharmacist and have been asked by the cardiology clinic to check his electrolytes one week after commencing. What is the most common risk associated with spironolactone?

☐A Hyperkalaemia
☐B Hypernatraemia
☐C Hypokalaemia
☐D Hyponatraemia
☐E Hypophosphataemia

299 Ms AL, an 82-year-old woman, has been struggling to swallow her citalopram 20mg tablets. She is currently on a dose of 20mg daily. The nursing home that she resides in are asking for an oral solution or a dissolvable tablet. You know that oral drops are available as citalopram 40mg/ml. 4 oral drops (8 mg) is equivalent in therapeutic effect to 10 mg tablet. How many drops are needed to ensure that the patient receives the correct dose?

☐A 0.5
☐B 4
☐C 8
☐D 16
☐E 18

300 What schedule of drug are pharmacists not allowed to be in possession of when acting in their capacity as a pharmacist?

☐A Schedule 1
☐B Schedule 2
☐C Schedule 3
☐D Schedule 4
☐E Schedule 5

Calculations

301 A 65-year-old male has been prescribed mitoxantrone to treat acute myeloid leukaemia. He has been prescribed a dose of 15mg/m2 daily for 7 days. The patient weighs 55kg and is 1.8m tall. Mitoxantrone is available as 10mg vials. How many vials are needed to complete the full course?

$$\text{BSA (m}^2) = \sqrt{\frac{\text{Ht (Cm)x Wt (kg)}}{3600}}$$

302 A 10-year-old female child has a weeping infected wound. The child has been prescribed potassium permanganate solution 1 in 4000. This product is prepared from a stock solution of 50 times this strength. How much potassium permanganate stock solution will be needed if the child uses 200ml of the diluted solution twice a day for 7 days? Give your answer to 3 decimal places in litres.

303 You have been asked to prepare 25 suppositories with each containing 40mg of magnesium sulphate in theobroma oil base. Each suppository will be made to a 300mg mould. You are required to make a surplus of 20% to account for any loss during production. Given that the displacement value of magnesium sulphate in theobroma oil base is 2, how much base will be required? Give your answer to 1 decimal place in grams.

304 You are working as a PCN pharmacist in collaboration with the local CCG on cost saving projects. You are reviewing the use of Drug Y and Drug Z as these cost less than Drug X at an equivalent dose. Costs are shown below:

Drug	Cost	Dose
Drug X	£34.55/28	1 tablet OD
Drug Y	£32.90/28	1 tablet OD
Drug Z	£31.95/28	1 tablet OD

You have reviewed 30 patients who are prescribed Drug X and of those patients, 90% are suitable to be switched to Drug Z. The practice has a repeat prescribing policy of 30 days treatment of prescription. What is the total saving for 3 repeats assuming all the eligible patients switch to using Drug Z? Give your answer to the nearest £10.

305 An 80-year-old male patient requests and manages his own medication. After starting some new medication, he now must order his prescriptions several times a month because the quantity and due dates are out of sync. You are a practice pharmacist and decide to synchronise all his medication together so that the prescription needs to be ordered just once a month, instead of several times a month.

	Strength	Dose	Days left of treatment
Atorvastatin	40 mg	Take ONE at night	15
Furosemide	20 mg	Take TWO in the morning & ONE at lunch time	8
Levothyroxine	25 mcg	Take ONE in the morning	26
Levothyroxine	50 mcg	Take ONE in the morning	26
Metformin	500 mg	Take ONE daily	28
Pioglitazone	15 mg	Take ONE daily	5
Ramipril	10 mg	Take ONE daily	13

How many additional Furosemide 20mg tablets should be prescribed to synchronise the patient's medications?

306 You receive the following prescription for a 12-year-old child weighing 40kg for the management of Guillain-Barré syndrome. How long will it take to complete the whole infusion if it was infused at the prescribed rate?

Today's date	Immunoglobulin 10% 0.8g/kg	0.8ml/kg/hr for 30 mins then 1.2ml/kg/hr for 40 mins then 1.8ml/kg/hr for 50 mins then 3ml/kg/hr for the remainder of the infusion	Doctor D.

307 A 65-year-old male has been prescribed ketorolac eye drops for the treatment of post operative pain and inflammation associated with a cataract surgery (for his left eye). He has been instructed to 'instil ONE drop into the affected eye three times a day starting one day prior to surgery, continue on the day of the surgery and for the first two weeks' of the postoperative period. An additional drop should be administered 15 to 60 minutes prior to surgery. Ketorolac 1mg/ml eye drop: 20 drops is equivalent to 1ml. Available as 3ml bottle. Calculate the volume in millilitres that will remain in the bottle after following the prescriber's instruction (assuming all drops were given). Give your answer to 2 decimal places.

308 A 68-years-old man has a medical history of Crohn's disease. He currently has a double stoma and has been advised to take Dioralyte at a dose of 20 sachets a day in divided doses. The atomic mass of sodium is 23 and the atomic mass of chloride is 35.5. Each sachet contains 3 mmol of sodium chloride. The recommended daily intake of sodium chloride is 6g. What percentage of the sodium chloride recommended daily allowance will the patient receive from the sachets if taken as directed? Give your answer to 1 decimal place.

309 A 60-year-old man weighing 88kg is 5 foot 6 inches (2.81 m2) tall. The patient has a complicated skin infection and has been prescribed IV vancomycin as advised by microbiology. An initial loading dose was administered, and you have been asked to calculate the patient's renal function*. His serum creatinine is 138 micromol/litre.

*When using Vancomycin the renal function should be calculated using the patients ideal body weight (IBW) if the BMI is >30.
- IBW Male (kg) = 50 + (2.3 x number of inches above 5 ft in height)
- IBW Female (kg) = 45.5 (2.3 x number of inches above 5 ft in height)
Constant: 1.23 for men; 1.04 for women
Calculate the renal function of the patient. Give your answer to 1 decimal place.

$$CrCl \ (ml/min) = \frac{(140 - Age) \times (Weight \ in \ kg) \times Constant}{Serum \ creatinine \ (micromol/L)}$$

310 A 16-year-old female is taking drug Z to manage an autoimmune disease. According to the SmPC the half-life of drug Z is 4 hours. The initial plasma level of the drug after a single dose was 4,480mg/L. The plasma level is now 4,375 microgram/L. How many minutes have passed since the initial dose?

311 Ms PA, a 42-year-old Caucasian woman, has had a flare up of psoriatic arthritis. The rheumatologist has started her on prednisolone tablets at a dose of 15mg daily, they have requested that she reduces her prednisolone by 2.5mg tablets every two weeks until stop. They have given her a two-week supply and requested that we arrange the rest. The rheumatologist has requested that we give the patient 2.5mg tablets only so to avoid confusion for the patient. How many 2.5mg tablets are needed to complete the course for this patient?

312 Baby SA, a 6-month-year old, has been prescribed antibiotics at a dose of 30mg/kg three times a day for 5 days. The strength of the suspension is 250mg in 5mls.
Baby SA weight: 7.5kg.
How many mls would baby SA be taking at each dose? Give your answer to 1 decimal place.

313 Mr PD an 82-year-old Asian man has been diagnosed with pancreatic cancer and is palliative. The Macmillan nurse has requested to change his Zomorph 30mg twice a day to Oxycontin. Using the table below what is the most appropriate daily dose for conversion? Please supply the strength and dose needed.

	Equivalent dose to 10mg oral morphine
Codeine phosphate	100mg
Dihydrocodeine	100mg
Hydromorphone	2mg
Methadone	*
Morphine	10mg
Oxycodone	6.6mg
Tapentadol	25mg
Tramadol	100mg

314 Miss CM, a 31-year-old Caucasian woman, is requesting norethisterone 5mg tablet for the postponement of menstruation as she is due to go away. She is going away from the 20th April – 1st May and her expected onset of her period is on the 21st April. She advises that she doesn't mind coming on any time on or after the 2nd May. You check the BNF and the dose is as follows:

> Postponement of menstruation
> By mouth
> For Females of childbearing potential
> 5 mg 3 times a day, to be started 3 days before expected onset (menstruation occurs 2–3 days after stopping).

What is the maximum number of 5mg norethisterone tablets that the patient requires for the whole course?

315 Mrs LA, a 58-year-old woman, is currently on Priadel® 400mg daily (lithium carbonate), during a recent SALT assessment they have requested to change her tablets to oral solution. The oral solution that is available is Priadel 520mg/5ml liquid (lithium citrate tetrahydrate). The BNF extract has been supplied. https://bnf.nice.org.uk/drugs/lithium-citrate/#indicationsAndDoses
What is the total daily dose in ml of Priadel 520mg/5ml that equates to taking Priadel 400mg daily tablet (give answer to the nearest ml)?

316 Mr AR, a 92-year-old Asian man, has been advised to take 400iu vitamin D a day. He is currently being prescribed Fultium D3 drops 2740iu/ml. There are 41 drops in 1ml. In order to get 400iu of vitamin D daily how many drops will the patient need to take?

317 Mrs SW, a 72-year-old woman, with COPD is taking carbocisteine capsules at 0.375g three times a day. She is currently struggling to swallow the capsules whole and is requesting if we can prescribe an oral solution? The oral solution is available as carbocisteine 250mg/5ml. How many ml will the patient need to cover a month's course (28 days)?

318 Mr AL, an 89-year-old man, has come into hospital with aspiration pneumonia. He requires his tablets to be converted to oral solution. He is currently on digoxin 125mcg daily.
Digoxin tablets have a bioavailability of 0.7
Digoxin oral solution has a bioavailability of 0.8
The oral solution is available as 50mcg/ml – how many ml should be given to Mr AL daily?

319 Mr FA a 45-year-old man is to receive 500ml of dextrose 5% over 4 hours. The set that it is given through delivers at 20 drops/ml. Calculate the required drip rate in drops/min.

320 Mrs OL, an 88-year-old woman, is currently NBM, she is experiencing great pain and the doctor decides to give her paracetamol as an intravenous infusion. Mrs OL weighs 48kg. The BNF extract is supplied.
https://bnf.nice.org.uk/drugs/paracetamol/
How many ml of solution will be infused in each dose IV if the amps available are at a dose of 1g/10ml? Give your answer to one decimal place.

Questions 321-325 require the use of the Cockcroft-Gault Equation.
Using the Cockcroft-Gault Equation which is
For women multiply the result of calculation by 0.85.

$$\text{Creatinine clearance} = \frac{((140 - \text{age in years}) \times (\text{weight in kg}) \times 1.23)}{(\text{serum creatinine in micromol/L})}$$

For 321 supply your answer to one decimal place
For 322, 323 and 325 supply your answer to the nearest whole number

Question	Age	Weight (kg)	Gender	Serum Creatinine (mmol/l)	Creatinine Clearance
321	79	65	Female	264	
322		81	Male	196	29.9
323	67		Male	81	85.4
324	61	54		288	15.4
325	54	79	Male		109.9

326 Mrs RG (age 77 years) has been taking prednisolone 5mg for the past 6 months for her polymyalgia rheumatica. She was advised by her rheumatologist to start weaning her dose down following a month of no symptoms. She contacts you to arrange a prescription for the correct quantity to be able to do this. Her weaning protocol is to wean by 1mg every 4 weeks and then stop and she wants to start weaning in four weeks time. What quantity of prednisolone 1mg tablets will be required to fulfil the prescription?

327 Mr MK (65 years) has been started on Humulin M3 Kwikpen 100units/ml suspension for injection following a type 2 diabetes review. His dose has been gradually titrated and he has been advised to remain on this dose until the next review and repeat HbA1C check is due in 3 months. This dose is 10 units in the morning and 12 units in the evening. Each pre-filled pen contains 3ml of biphasic isophane insulin. How many pens does Mr MK need for a one month (28 days) supply?

328 Mrs BS (62 years) is applying Oestrogel 0.06% gel as the product of choice for her hormonal replacement therapy. Recently the dose for her estradiol has been increased to 3mg once daily. Each pump delivers 1.25g of gel which contains 0.75mg of estradiol. The gel is available as a pack of 80g. She requests that she is prescribed enough to last her 2 months as she pays for her prescription. How many packs does Mrs BS need to be prescribed?

329 Mr MH (28 years) has been prescribed some Eumovate (clobetasone 0.05%) cream to treat a flare up of his eczema. His symptoms are confined only to his arms and so the GP has prescribed a 30gram tube. How much clobetasone is in the 30gram tube?

330 You receive a letter from Ms SY's endocrinologist, advising that Ms SY should reduce her dose of prednisolone by 1mg every 4 days. She is currently taking 26mg daily. How many 1mg and 5mg tablets do you need to prescribe for the next 4 weeks (28 days)?

331 You are a hospital pharmacist working on the paediatric ward. Baby ZQ (6 months) is to be initiated on furosemide slow IV infusion. Baby weight = 4.5kg. The highest possible initial dose according to weight is to be started. 20mg/2ml injections are available on the ward. Furosemide BNF insert has been provided https://bnfc.nice.org.uk/drugs/furosemide/ What is the rate per dose? Please provide the answer ml/hourly rate to 3 decimal places.

332 Mr RF (63 years) is being discharged from hospital following his exacerbation of COPD. You are the respiratory pharmacist working on the ward and are asked to prepare medication for Mr RF's discharge. Ipratropium nebules 250mcg/ml are prescribed at 250mcg four times daily. How many packs (pack size 20 nebules) will be needed to complete a two week take home medicine prescription?

333 You are a hospital pharmacist working in the outpatients department. Mr VL (65 years) has been reviewed by the ENT specialist. He has been prescribed Maxidex eye drops 1 drop to the left eye 6 times a day for 28 days. How many 5ml bottles will be needed to fulfil the prescription? The rheumatologist has asked you to prescribe a reduced course of prednisolone for your patient. They are currently taking 30mg daily and should reduce by 5mg every fortnight to a maintenance dose of 5mg daily. How many 5mg tablets are required for the next 12 weeks?

334 You are working on some cost saving audits in your GP Practice. One of your responsibilities is to make savings to the practice drug budget. 17 patients are prescribed pregabalin 150mg caps TWO twice daily. Switching these patients to pregabalin 300mg ONE twice daily can provide significant cost savings for the practice. If these patients are all suitable to switch, how much will you save the practice in 1 year (work out to 364 days)? Give your answer to the nearest ten pounds.

Pregabalin 150mg caps x 56 = £64.40
Pregabalin 300mg caps x 56 = £64.40

336 You are a primary care pharmacist and have received a letter from the opioid dependence clinic. The clinic has reviewed the patient and has asked the surgery to take over the prescribing of buprenorphine tablets. The patient's new dose is buprenorphine 1.6mg daily. You have called the

patients pharmacy and all strengths are out of stock apart from 0.4mg tablets. How many tablets do you need to supply a 7-day prescription?

337 The junior doctor on the acute admissions ward asks for your help with the prescribing of 'dual sachets' of Gaviscon for a 1-year-old child. The child's weight is 5kg and the doctor wants to ensure the child gets the correct amount at each bottle feed. The doctor isn't sure how to calculate this, as he says they come as 'dual sachets' and wants you work it out. The child has 3 bottle feeds in 24 hours. Calculate how many sachets of Gaviscon you will prescribe for 4 weeks. https://www.medicines.org.uk/emc/product/6581/smpc

338 Master RD is 7 years old and weighs 23.2kg. He has recently come out of hospital following a seizure. The discharge summary asks you to add carbamazepine liquid to the patient's repeat prescriptions. The doctor wants Master RD to start on 2.5mg/kg twice daily for the first 7 days, then increase the dose by 2.5mg/kg every 7 days for the next two weeks. At this point he will be reviewed with the paediatrics team at hospital. Carbamazepine 100mg/5ml is available. What volume of liquid will you need to cover the course? Give your answer to the nearest ml.

339 Baby X is 3 years and 7 months old. She has been diagnosed with multiple sclerosis. You have been sent a task from the speech and language therapy (SALT) team to add Thick and Easy clear powder to her regular repeat prescription. The SALT team have told you that she is currently IDDSI level 2 and using 2 scoops per 200mls, 5 times a day. The tin contains 126g of powder and 1 scoop size is 1.4g. How much Thick and Easy will need prescribing every 28 days?

340 You are a hospital pharmacist working on the female surgical ward. A patient has been admitted for elective surgery. She is being treated for epilepsy with carbamazepine and is currently nil by mouth. Her medication on admission includes carbamazepine prolonged release tablets 400 mg twice daily. You decide to switch to suppositories which will be administered four times a day. What strength suppository is required for each individual dose? Guidance is provided: https://www.medicines.org.uk/emc/product/12866/smpc#gref

341 You are a quality control pharmacist working for a large wholesaling unit that deals with unlicensed medication supplies. You have been asked to help regarding the preparation of a new medicine. You need to prepare 250mg of the drug at a concentration of 3mg/ml. The displacement value is 0.5ml/50mg. What volume of diluent is required in order to produce the final concentration? Give your answer to one decimal place.

342 You are a pharmacist working in a specialised unit. You have been asked to prepare 24 suppositories in a 2g mould with each suppository containing 0.08g of bismuth subgallate. Calculate the total amount (grams) of base that you require if the displacement value of bismuth subgallate is 2.6. Give your answer to two decimal places.

343 You have a stock solution of drug Z with a concentration of 10% w/v. Drug Z is used as an antiseptic wash at a concentration of 0.475% w/v. You receive a request to supply 500ml of a solution of intermediate strength so that the patient will dilute this solution 1 in 20 in order for them to use it accurately. What is the concentration, % w/v, of the intermediate solution? Give your answer to one decimal place?

344 You are a hospital pharmacist working on the gynaecology ward. Miss KF (33 years) is 28 weeks pregnant, and the consultant has requested Ferinject IV infusion is prescribed for this patient with a view to correct levels as soon as possible. The consultant has requested Miss KF is on the maximum dose. You review her medical notes:

Hb = <6.2mmol/l
Weight = 62kg

You have access to the SPC: https://www.medicines.org.uk/emc/product/5910/smpc#gref

What volume of Ferinject is needed for Mrs KF's initial dose?

345 You are asked to make a chlorhexidine stock solution for disinfection. What strength of chlorhexidine solution (mg/mL) do you need to prepare

so that when 5 mL is diluted to 100 mL it provides a final concentration of 0.06%?

346 You are a paediatric pharmacist working on the neonatal ward. Baby PL (2 weeks old, weighing 3 kg) is prescribed midazolam following his febrile convulsions. Midazolam 100mg/50ml solution for infusion is available. What is the rate of the continuous infusion following his initial dose? Give the answer to ml/min to 4 decimal places. A BNF extract has been supplied: https://bnfc.nice.org.uk/drug/midazolam.html#indicationsAndDoses

347 Mr BM (5 years, weighing 17.4kg) has been diagnosed with a severe complicated urinary tract infection. You are a hospital pharmacist and discuss the case with microbiology. They suggest treatment dose of fosfomycin. They recommend 300mg/kg daily in 3 divided doses. You have access to the 2g vials. The nurse asks you what volume of reconstituted fosfomycin vials should be drawn up for each dose? Give your answer to 1 decimal place. The SPC is available to you: https://www.medicines.org.uk/emc/product/11249/smpc#gref

348 You receive a prescription for Master AR (age 5 years) for 500g of coal tar with zinc oxide paste BP. You are unable to source it and decide to prepare extemporaneously. You allow for 10% excess. How much zinc oxide is needed? Give your answer in milligrams. https://bnf.nice.org.uk/drug/coal-tar-with-zinc-oxide.html#prescribingAndDispensingInformations

349 Mrs LP (72 years) is prescribed potassium chloride 4.2g OD for the prevention of hypokalaemia. She will be receiving her dose via 600mg tablets. What weight in milligrams of potassium is in each dose? The molecular weights are potassium 39.1 and chloride 35.5. Give your answer to the nearest whole number in milligrams.

350 A 3-year-old child weighing 13.2kg is being treated for suspected pneumonia. The drug of choice is benzylpenicillin. The recommended dose is 25mg/kg every 6 hours. Benzylpenicillin 600mg/2ml vials are available to you. What volume in mls is needed for the daily dose? Give your answer to one decimal place.

351 You are working in an aseptics unit and have received a request to prepare 300ml of an oral solution which contains sodium bicarbonate 2mmol / 5ml. You have 8.4% sodium bicarbonate available. How many mls of the 8.4% solution will you need in order to prepare the request?
Mr Sodium bicarbonate = 84.

352 Master FL (age 8 years) is being initiated on lisinopril for hypertension. His weight is 23kg. What volume in mls will be needed at each dose? You have 5mg/5ml oral solution available. BNF extract: https://bnfc.nice.org.uk/drugs/lisinopril/
Give your answer to two decimal places.

353 A hospital pharmacist is reconstituting a vial of piperacillin sodium (2g vials). The vial is mixed with sterile water (10mls) for injection. The solution is then diluted by adding 50ml of 5% dextrose injection for administration by infusion. What is the final concentration of piperacillin sodium in the solution? Give you answer in mg/ml.

354 Mr BC is admitted onto the acute admissions ward due to resistant oedema. The consultant has prescribed IV furosemide 100mg stat. You have 20mg/2ml ampoules available. The infusion is being given undiluted. What is the fastest rate that an infusion can be set at? https://bnf.nice.org.uk/drugs/furosemide/

355 Mrs LV has been admitted to the acute medical admissions ward with suspected digoxin toxicity. Blood tests are taken and her serum digoxin level is currently 6.3 mcg/L. The consultant is wanting to start DigiFab. You have access to the SPC: https://digifab.health/getmedia/6f38d7ed-1832-4b7d-863a-9c71905e4d02/SmPC_DigiFab_Dec17.pdf
Mrs LV's weight on admission is 63.9 kg. What number of 40mg vials is needed?

356 You receive the following request 'send 400mL benzalkonium chloride solution which when diluted 1 in 50 produces a 1 in 250 solution.' You have access to 40% w/v benzalkonium chloride available. What volume of this concentrate is needed to fulfil your request? Give your answer to the nearest whole mL.

357 You are an aseptics pharmacist working in an outpatients unit. A stock solution of chlorhexidine acetate is available in 1L bottles at a concentration of 0.06% w/v. How many millilitres of purified water is required to be added to 20ml of the stock solution to prepare a 20ppm solution of chlorhexidine acetate for use as a burns dressing for the skin? Give your answer to the nearest whole millilitre.

358 Mr GH (53-years-old) is diagnosed with testicular cancer. You are a hospital pharmacist working on the oncology ward. Mr GH is initiated on etoposide. The consultant would like the patient to receive one treatment course (using the higher limit of the dosing range). Mr GH weighs 72 kg and is 195 cm tall. What is the total amount of 50mg capsules needed for the full course? BNF extract: https://bnf.nice.org.uk/drugs/etoposide/

$$BSA \ (m^2) = \sqrt{\frac{Ht \ (Cm) x \ Wt \ (kg)}{3600}}$$

359 You are a pharmacist working in a manufacturing unit. You have been asked to make a batch of 10 suppositories, each containing 15 mg of hydrocortisone in a theobroma oil base. The final weight of each suppository is 2g and you should make a 10% excess. The displacement value of hydrocortisone in theobroma oil is 1.5. How much theobroma oil do you require? Give you answer to one decimal place.

360 Mr KG (88 years) is a palliative care patient. He has been prescribed diamorphine slow intravenous injection 2.5mg every four hours PRN. If Mr KG were to take the max dose in 24 hours, how many 10mg ampoules will be required over one week?

Further questions

The next five questions (361-365) are based on the same list of options, but different scenarios. Each option may be used once, more than once, or not at all.

Theme: Headache

- ☐ **A** Cluster headache
- ☐ **B** Medication overuse headache
- ☐ **C** Migraine with aura
- ☐ **D** Migraine without aura
- ☐ **E** Side effect of medication
- ☐ **F** Sinusitis
- ☐ **G** Subarachnoid haemorrhage
- ☐ **H** Tension headache

361 A 51-year-old male presents with a severe unilateral headache which lasts for approximately 20 minutes and generally occurs at the same time of day. The trigger is usually when he is physically exerted. The headache is frontal and also associated with flushing.

362 A 28-year-old female presents with a bilateral pulsating headache. This is usually triggered by eating chocolate or skipping meals. The pain is quite severe and also associated with photosensitivity, visual disturbances and vomiting.

363 A 58-year-old woman presents to the community pharmacy with the following symptoms: Sudden onset thunderclap headache and severe pain at the back of the head within 5 minutes.

364 A 32-year-old male presents with frequent headaches that last between 30mins-7 days. He has a highly stressful job. The headache is bilateral with a 'pressing feeling' and moderate intensity in pain. There is no nausea or vomiting associated.

365 A 51-year-old patient who was recently started on amlodipine 5mg for the management of her hypertension. She has a history of migraines. The headache she describes is bilateral and non-pulsating.

The next five questions (366-370) are based on the same list of options, but different scenarios. Each option may be used once, more than once, or not at all.

Theme: Narrow therapeutic index drugs

 □ A Amiodarone
 □ B Carbamazepine
 □ C Digoxin
 □ D Lithium
 □ E Phenobarbitol
 □ F Phenytoin
 □ G Theophylline
 □ H Warfarin

366 The plasma drug concentration for optimum response is 4-12mg/litre.

367 Patients should be advised to be able to recognise signs and symptoms of blood, liver and skin disorders such as fever, rash, mouth ulcer, bruising or bleeding developing.

368 Patients should be advised on the potential effects on driving and performing skilled tasks due to the risks of corneal microdeposits which is associated with blurred vision.

369 Patients should be advised to shield skin from sunlight during treatment and for several months after discontinuation. Sunscreen is also recommended.

370 Patients should be advised to maintain adequate fluid intake and keep their diet consistent with regards to sodium intake as a change can lead to altered drug levels.

371 You are a community pharmacist and you receive a referral through the local GP practice for MR FH's (age 23) for his sinusitis. The referral is via the community pharmacy consultation services. Which of the following statements regarding the service is correct?

   □ A NHS England does not need to be notified when a pharmacy delivers this service
   □ B Referrals for emergency supply of medication are not expected
   □ C The CPCS can expect referrals from NHS 111
   □ D This is a referral pathway for all medical conditions
   □ E This is an example of an enhanced pharmacy service

372 A 33-year-old patient is admitted into hospital with a flare up of ulcerative colitis. You are writing up the drug chart for this patient and note she will require venous thromboembolism prophylaxis (VTE). Which of the following is a correct statement regarding dalteparin?

   □ A Dose reduction is not usually required in patients with renal impairment
   □ B Platelet counts should ideally be checked prior to treatment dose
   □ C Routine monitoring of anti-factor Xa levels is recommended
   □ D The usual dose is given via intravenous injection
   □ E When checking anti-factor Xa levels for DVT/ PE treatment – levels should be checked 12 hours post dose

373 Mr GS (54-year-old male) presents to the community pharmacy complaining about his red eye. The red eye started one day ago. You examine the eye and note you may need to refer this patient. Which of the following symptoms would require a referral to the GP?

   □ A Excessive watery discharge
   □ B Irregular pupil size
   □ C Purulent discharge from the eye
   □ D Red eye
   □ E Sore eye

374 You are a community pharmacist, and your regular patient Mr TV (62 years) has been initiated on rivaroxaban 15mg OD. You deem it appropriate to undertake a 'new medicines service' (NMS). Which of the following statements is correct regarding the NMS service?

☐ **A** Rivaroxaban would not fall under a category for the NMS service
☐ **B** The NMS service covers patients with osteoporosis
☐ **C** The NMS service is an example of an Enhanced Service
☐ **D** There is no reimbursement to the pharmacy for this service
☐ **E** The service can generally be provided if the formulation of drug changes for the patient

The next five questions (375-379) are based on the same list of options, but different scenarios. Each option may be used once, more than once, or not at all.

Theme: Cardiovascular medication

☐ **A** Apixaban
☐ **B** Aspirin
☐ **C** Clopidogrel
☐ **D** Enoxaparin
☐ **E** Fondaparinux
☐ **F** Rivaroxaban
☐ **G** Ticagrelor
☐ **H** Warfarin

375 Mr BH (72 years) is admitted onto the acute stroke ward due to a transient ischaemic attack. The consultant prescribes this medication long term post discharge.

376 Mr DP (28 years) has been diagnosed with a spontaneous DVT. Mr DP chooses this treatment as it works well with his lifestyle. The course is for six months, the dosing is once daily and no routine monitoring is needed.

377 Mrs WP (75 years) is initiated on this medication after a diagnosis of atrial fibrillation. The drug will need the following routine monitoring: weight, creatinine and age.

378 Miss KC (29 years) requires anithrombotic treatment for prevention of VTE during her inpatient stay on the cardiovascular ward. This drug is selected as she is vegan and it is a synthetic based drug (not derived from animal tissue).

379 Mrs LP (54 years) has been initiated on this medication for treatment of pulmonary embolism. When counselling you advise her to report any painful skin rashes due to the risk of calciphylaxis.

380 Mr FB (54 years) is under the care of the heart failure team due to a new diagnosis. You manage your diabetic clinics within an outpatient hospital setting. Mr FB is currently prescribed the following: ramipril 2.5mg OD, atorvastatin 80mg OD, metformin 1g BD, gliclazide 40mg BD, linagliptin 5mg OD, clopidogrel 75mg OD, tiotropium 18cg inh 1 OD, salbutamol 100mcg OD, relvar 92/22 Inh 1 OD. The heart failure nurses have requested that he should be initiated on bisoprolol 2.5mg OD for the long-term management of his heart failure. Which of the following is a correct statement regarding the management plan?

- ☐ A Bisoprolol dose is too low, it needs to be 5mg OD
- ☐ B Bisoprolol is not appropriate, amend to alternative betablocker
- ☐ C Counsel patient on the risks of hypoglycaemia and hyperglycaemia
- ☐ D Counsel patient on the risks of rebound hypotension when taking this medication
- ☐ E Counsel patient on the risks of taking betablockers with his current comorbidities and suggest that this drug should not be prescribed

381 Mrs GB (71 years) visits the community pharmacy complaining of muscular aches and pains. You check your PMR and note that she was recently initiated on a medication which may be the cause. Mrs GB is referred to the GP and she is diagnosed with rhabdomyolysis. Which of the following is the most likely drug cause?

- ☐ A Apixaban
- ☐ B Pravastatin
- ☐ C Rivaroxaban
- ☐ D Sulfasalazine
- ☐ E Ursodeoxycholic acid

382 Mrs LF (64 years) has her annual health review and the nurse notes she may be eligible for statin medication. Mrs LF has a past medical history of hysterectomy and hypothyroidism. You are the community pharmacist working on site and help the practice nurse calculate the QRISK3 score. The score is worked out at 15%. Mrs LF's recent cholesterol level was 4.5. Which of the following statements is correct?

    ☐ A The cholesterol level is high thus the patient requires a statin after a lifestyle intervention/discussion

    ☐ B The cholesterol level is low thus the patient does not require a statin

    ☐ C The QRISK score is low and the patient should not be prescribed a statin

    ☐ D The QRISK score is raised and the patient is eligible for a statin after a lifestyle intervention/discussion

    ☐ E The QRISK score is within the recommended range

The next five questions (383-387) are based on the same list of options, but different scenarios. Each option may be used once, more than once, or not at all.

Theme: Side effects to medication

    ☐ A Atenolol
    ☐ B Atorvastatin
    ☐ C Bisoprolol
    ☐ D Carbimazole
    ☐ E Metronidazole
    ☐ F Perindopril
    ☐ G Phenytoin
    ☐ H Thiamine

383 Mr BP (52 years) is initiated on this medication however you advise the GP against the prescribing of this as you are aware Mr BP has previously had angioedema.

384 Mrs NN (42 years) is initiated on this medication for her angina after complaining of nightmares with her previous medication.

385 Mr GJ (68 years) is initiated on this medication and you advise against drinking grapefruit juice due to an interaction.

386 Mrs AD (46 years) is prescribed this medication and you advise against drinking alcohol due to the risk of an interaction.

387 Mr PL (65 years) is prescribed this medication following endocrine review. You advise Mr PL to monitor for any sore throats that may occur whilst taking this medication.

388 Mr SA (22 years) visits your community pharmacy wishing to discuss the options for smoking cessation. He has been advised by his best friend that he was given a tablet which 'worked wonders with his cravings'. Mr SA is hoping that he is able to buy these tablets today to help him quit smoking. What is the most appropriate management plan?

☐ A Advise Mr SA that a similar table is usually offered first line by the GP
☐ B Advise Mr SA that combination NRT or varenicline have all been shown to be effective
☐ C Advise Mr SA that this tablet does not exist
☐ D Advise Mr SA to start combination NRT
☐ E All of the above

389 You are a manager of a community pharmacy in a busy inner-city practice. You decide to opt for the smoking cessation service in order to support your patients. Which of the following is CORRECT about the service?

☐ A Patients can self-refer for this service
☐ B People aged 16 years and older who have started treatment for tobacco dependence in hospital and have chosen to continue their treatment in community pharmacy after discharge are eligible
☐ C This is an enhanced service
☐ D This service does not include pregnant patients
☐ E To provide the service, contractors must have a carbon monoxide (CO) monitor

390 Miss FP (11 years old) presents to the community pharmacy with a prescription for her acne medication. Which of the following should be avoided?

☐ A Adapalene
☐ B Azelaic acid
☐ C Benzoyl peroxide
☐ D Lymecycline
☐ E Trimethoprim

Case based discussions

The following are some case studies to help you prepare your learning/revision

391 Travel health:

Miss TC (25 years) visits your community pharmacy informing you that she is planning on travelling to South Africa for 6 months. She is unsure if she needs malaria prophylaxis and asks you for your advice.

392 Smoking Cessation:

Mr AS (35 years) visits the community pharmacy and informs you that is wanting to quit smoking. He would like advice regarding the various options available to him.

393 Post discharge – myocardial infarction:

Mr HA (64 years) is discharged from the hospital. He had nil medical history prior to admission and had a sudden heart attack. He is initiated on multiple new medication and would like to discuss all the medication with you.

394 Inpatient prescription for gentamicin:

Mr IU (58 years) is to be prescribed IV gentamicin as part of 'blind therapy' for an undiagnosed serious infection on a vascular word. The nurse asks for your advice regarding dosing regime and also monitoring. Discuss the options for treatment and monitoring needed.

395 Emergency contraception in a community pharmacy setting:

Miss LP (25 years) visits the community pharmacy and would like to buy the emergency contraceptive pill. She usually takes Yasmin 1 OD but has missed a few days so is unsure if the morning after pill will be indicated.

396 Hormonal replacement therapy review in primary care:

Miss LG (58 years) is due an annual review of her HRT medication, she currently uses an evorel conti patch. What will you discuss at the review?

397 Sore throat presentation in the community pharmacy:

Mr FZ (age 28 years) visits the community pharmacy to discuss a painful sore throat which developed 4 days ago. His throat is sore, painful and he is struggling to swallow due to the pain. Mr FZ is hoping for some pain relief to help with his sore throat.

398 Sumatriptan supply in the community pharmacy:

Mr PL (29 years) would like to buy a table to help relieve his migraine. He has heard about sumatriptan. He has not been diagnosed by the doctor in the past. Can sumatriptan be supplied?

399 Dandruff management:

Miss KL (5 years) is brought into the pharmacy with mum due to concerns regarding dandruff. On examination the 'dandruff' is headlice. They would like to purchase something over the counter to treat the lice.

400 Outpatient prescription for darbepoetin alfa:

Mrs LP (68 years) is a renal dialysis patient who has recently been prescribed darbepoetin alfa. You are the pharmacist working in the outpatient's dispensary. You clinically check the prescription.

High weighted answers

1   **A - Amlodipine**
ACE are generally less effective as monotherapy in African Caribbean patients because of the tendency towards a low renin state, a lower cardiac output, and an increased peripheral resistance.
https://www.nice.org.uk/guidance/ng136

2   **E - Ramipril**
One of the more common side effects of ACE inhibitors is a persistent dry cough. The same activity that allows ACE inhibitors to lower blood pressure can cause other substances, like bradykinin, to accumulate in the airways. This can trigger airway inflammation and coughing in some people.
https://bnf.nice.org.uk/drugs/ramipril/#side-effects

3   **D - losartan**
A cough occurs in about 15% of people taking an ACE inhibitor and may occur at any time after starting treatment. If the cough is troublesome (for example, it prevents the person from sleeping) and other causes have been ruled out, consider switching to an angiotensin-II receptor blocker.
https://cks.nice.org.uk/topics/hypertension/prescribing-information/angiotensin-converting-enzyme-inhibitors/

4   **A - Amlodipine**
Ankle swelling is a common, often problematic adverse effect for patients on CCB and this may affect compliance. It is due to changes in capillary pressure leading to leakage into interstitial areas, rather than due to water retention.
https://pharmaceutical-journal.com/article/ld/your-patient-has-swollen-ankles-linked-with-the-use-of-calcium-channel-blockers

5   **C - Indapamide**

As per NHS guidelines, for a patient currently on ACE and CCB, the next stage is a thiazide like diuretic. Patients' amlodipine could be increased to 10mg OD however given the patients BMI, there is an increased risk of ankle swelling. Add in thiazide like diuretic and monitor the response.
https://www.nice.org.uk/guidance/ng136/chapter/Recommendations# choosing-antihypertensive-drug-treatment-for-people-with-or-without- type-2-diabetes

6   **C - Potassium is ≤4.5**

Only prescribe spironolactone for people whose blood potassium level is 4.5 mmol/l or lower. There is an increased risk of hyperkalaemia in patients over 4.5.
https://bnf.nice.org.uk/drugs/spironolactone/

7   **D - The GP can prescribe the sodium valproate providing the GP discusses pregnancy risks and ensures if the patient is sexually active, that contraception is in place to prevent pregnancy**

The GP cannot prescribe the sodium valproate unless the neurologist feels that there is no effective alternative option and signs the patient up to the pregnancy prevention programme, explaining and making the patient aware of the risks. Note if the patient does decide to become pregnant, sodium valproate then becomes contraindicated.
https://www.gov.uk/drug-safety-update/valproate-pregnancy-prevention- programme-actions-required-now-from-gps-specialists-and-dispensers

8   **C - Advise GP that zopiclone is only for short-term use for up to 4 weeks**

Avoid prolonged use of zopiclone as there is a risk of tolerance and withdrawal symptoms
https://bnf.nice.org.uk/drugs/zopiclone/

9   **E - The dose of escitalopram should be reduced to 10mg daily in patients older than 65**

The dose of escitalopram should be reduced to 10mg daily in patients older than 65 as escitalopram is associated with dose-dependent QT interval prolongation.
https://www.gov.uk/drug-safety-update/citalopram-and-escitalopram-qt- interval-prolongation

10 **B - 0.4 – 1 mmol/L**
Samples should be taken 12 hours after the dose to achieve a serum-lithium concentration of 0.4–1 mmol/Litre. This is the lower end of the range for maintenance therapy and elderly patients.
https://bnf.nice.org.uk/drugs/lithium-carbonate/

11 **C - Advise the patient to see her GP immediately – it is likely that the medication she is taking is causing her symptoms**
The patient is presenting with symptoms that are concerning considering she is on carbamazepine. Patients, or their carers, should be told how to recognise signs of blood, liver, or skin disorders, and advised to seek immediate medical attention if symptoms such as fever, rash, mouth ulcers, bruising, or bleeding develop.
Note: the patient is on cimetidine which looks as though it is new based on the dosing. Cimetidine interacts with carbamazepine, increasing the concentration.
https://bnf.nice.org.uk/drugs/carbamazepine/#patient-and-carer-advice

12 **A - Amitriptyline**
The patient is likely experiencing anticholinergic syndrome, a side effect of amitriptyline.
https://bnfc.nice.org.uk/drugs/amitriptyline-hydrochloride/

13 **D - Codeine is suitable in children (under 18) who undergo the removal of tonsils or adenoids for the treatment of obstructive sleep apnoea**
Codeine is in fact contraindicated in all children (under 18 years) who undergo the removal of tonsils or adenoids for the treatment of obstructive sleep apnoea.
https://bnf.nice.org.uk/drugs/codeine-phosphate/

14 **A - Empagliflozin**
A review by the European Medicines Agency has concluded that serious, life-threatening, and fatal cases of diabetic ketoacidosis (DKA) have been reported rarely in patients taking an SGLT2 inhibitor.
https://bnf.nice.org.uk/drugs/empagliflozin/

15 C - Metformin

Metformin is used for the treatment of polycystic ovary syndrome but is not licensed for this indication.

https://bnf.nice.org.uk/drugs/metformin-hydrochloride/#unlicensed-use

16 B - Gliclazide

Gliclazide should be used with care in those with mild to moderate renal impairment because of the increased risk of hypoglycaemia. They should be avoided where possible in severe renal impairment.

https://bnf.nice.org.uk/treatment-summaries/type-2-diabetes/

17 E - Sitagliptin

Discontinue if symptoms of acute pancreatitis occur such as persistent, severe abdominal pain.

https://bnf.nice.org.uk/drugs/sitagliptin/

18 D - Pioglitazone

Incidence of heart failure is increased when pioglitazone is combined with insulin, especially in patients with predisposing factors, e.g. previous myocardial infarction.

https://bnf.nice.org.uk/drugs/pioglitazone

19 D - Abrupt withdrawal after a weeks' worth of prednisolone can lead to hypovolaemic shock

This is false because gradual withdrawal should be considered in patients who have received more than 40mg prednisolone or equivalent daily for more than a week. Also, abrupt withdrawal of prednisolone does not lead to hypovolaemic shock.

https://bnf.nice.org.uk/drugs/prednisolone/#treatment-cessation

20 C - Impetigo

Impetigo is red sores or blisters that burst leaving crusty, golden brown patches.

https://cks.nice.org.uk/topics/impetigo/diagnosis/clinical-features/

21 E - Vancomycin

Vancomycin is a narrow-spectrum bactericidal antibiotic used primarily for treatment of serious staphylococcal infections.

https://bnf.nice.org.uk/drugs/vancomycin/

22 **B - Doxycycline**

Doxycycline – patient is allergic to penicillin – as per guidelines.

Antibiotic treatment for adults ≥18 years (5–7 days treatment).

First-choice alternative: clarithromycin 500 mg b.d or doxycycline 200 mg on day 1, then 100 mg OD. In the cases of antibiotic choice, local guidance usually used, in this case D and E are more appropriate for urinary tract infections and A and C are not appropriate for patients with a penicillin allergy.

https://cks.nice.org.uk/topics/insect-bites-stings/

23 **C - *Helicobacter pylori***

Helicobacter pylori – eradication therapy. See BNF (two antibiotics and PPI cover for 2 weeks).

https://bnf.nice.org.uk/treatment-summaries/helicobacter-pylori-infection/

24 **A - 1st line treatment is chloramphenicol 0.5% eye drops – 1 drop 2 hourly for 2 days, reducing to 4 hourly as the infection improves for 7 days**

This is false because treatment should be continued for 48 hours after resolution of symptoms. Note: You should advise patients to see the GP if there is no improvement or worsening within 7 days as the patient may require fusidic eye drops and will need to be swabbed for a culture and sensitivity.

https://www.medicines.org.uk/emc/product/13182/smpc

25 **C - If the patient is taking frequent rescue packs they should be reviewed with the GP. The GP should review prescribing of rescue packs, review antibiotic choice including sputum cultures and sensitivities and consider if symptoms are masking anything more sinister like lung cancer**

It is not A because some exacerbations can be caused by viral infections and therefore rescue packs are not helpful in this context.

It is not B because co-amoxiclav contains penicillin and isn't appropriate for prescribing as a rescue pack.

It is not D because it is more than 3 issues in the last 12 months.

It is not E because the patient can have a rescue pack without sample, providing it isn't more than 3 issues per year.

ANSWERS

26 D - Nitrofurantoin

Nitrofurantoin is first line although borderline as it is contraindicated in patients with an eGFR <45ml/min. Since the patients eGFR is 46ml/min, it is appropriate to give nitrofurantoin for a short course. A, B and E contain penicillin. Fosfomycin is only advised. If a patient is penicillin allergic (anaphylaxis) and has poor renal function whereby other antibiotic options can't be used, then fosfomycin (prescribed as Monuril) 3g STAT once only can be given.

https://bnf.nice.org.uk/treatment-summaries/urinary-tract-infections/

27 C - Angiotensin receptor blockers (ARB)s

Avoid ARB's as these may also cause delayed angioedema.

https://www.nhs.uk/conditions/angioedema/causes/

28 C - Angiotensin receptor blockers (ARB)s

Unlike ACE inhibitors, they do not inhibit the breakdown of bradykinin and other kinins, and thus are less likely to cause the persistent dry cough which can complicate ACE inhibitor therapy.

https://bnf.nice.org.uk/treatment-summaries/drugs-affecting-the-renin-angiotensin-system/

29 G - Potassium sparing diuretics/mineralocorticoid receptor antagonists.

As per NICE guidance and stepwise management. The patient is currently already prescribed an ACE inhibitor and a beta-blocker.

https://www.nice.org.uk/guidance/ng106

30 F - Loop diuretics

Diuretics can exacerbate gout.

https://bnf.nice.org.uk/treatment-summaries/diuretics/

31 A - Advise her that it may take 2-3 weeks before she notices any improvement

SSRI's can take at least 2-3 weeks before any improvement is noticed, patients should be informed to persevere.

https://bnf.nice.org.uk/treatment-summaries/antidepressant-drugs/

32 **B - Citalopram above the dose of 20mg in the elderly is not appropriate**
Citalopram above the dose of 20mg in the elderly is not appropriate due to the risk of QT prolongation.
https://www.gov.uk/drug-safety-update/citalopram-and-escitalopram-qt-interval-prolongation

33 **D - Levonorgestrel intrauterine system**
Method of contraception should be highly effective.
https://bnf.nice.org.uk/treatment-summaries/contraceptives-hormonal/

34 **D - Take the morning dose and reduce the evening dose by 50%**
Guidance as per the International Diabetes Federation for adjustments for diabetic patients during the month of Ramadhan. This is based on the fact that this patient is on a long-acting insulin, without any administration of short acting insulin.
https://www.idf.org/our-activities/education/diabetes-and-ramadan.html

35 **D - Raised TSH and low T4**
It is most likely due to the symptoms provided by the patient. It is most likely a thyroid abnormality such as hypothyroidism. As per the BNF, NICE and the British Thyroid Association, hypothyroidism is diagnosed when TSH is raised and T4 is low.
Note: when TSH is raised and T4 normal, this is subclinical hypothyroidism and management depends on repeated tests. The GP would have ruled out low folate and ferritin as the FBC came back normal and thus this rules out anaemias.
https://bnf.nice.org.uk/treatment-summaries/hypothyroidism/

36 **C - Serum calcium levels**
To rule out excessive calcium levels.
https://bnf.nice.org.uk/drugs/colecalciferol/#sideEffects

37 **C - Desmopressin nasal spray**
Desmopressin is an analogue of vasopressin and can cause these side effects.
https://bnf.nice.org.uk/drugs/desmopressin/?msclkid=b07683d5ce5211eca37a2b62d3ecadb5#sideEffects

ANSWERS

38 **C - DEET dilutes sunscreen so apply SPF 30-50 first, then DEET at >20% concentration**
DEET reduces the protection provided by SPF15 sunscreen, according to several studies. When applying >33 percent dosages of DEET, sunscreen has not been demonstrated to reduce its effectiveness. PHE's 2015 recommendations state that sunscreen with an SPF of 30–50 should be applied first, followed by DEET. RED WHALE UK

39 **E – Shingles**
This is a classic example of a shingles presentation due to the rash type, location and symptoms described by the patient.
https://cks.nice.org.uk/topics/shingles/

40 **C – Erythromycin 500mg BD**
This is second line, the first line option is usually phenoxymethylpenicillin however the patient has had a rash previously.
https://bnf.nice.org.uk/drugs/erythromycin/

41 **E - Trimethoprim 200mg BD for 3 days**
Avoid nitrofurantoin due to low eGFR, 100mg is a low dose for trimethoprim, flucloxacillin not indicated.
https://cks.nice.org.uk/topics/urinary-tract-infection-lower-women/

42 **D - Propranolol**
Some beta-blockers are lipid soluble and some are water soluble. Water-soluble beta blockers (such as atenolol, celiprolol hydrochloride, nadolol, and sotalol hydrochloride) are less likely to enter the brain and may therefore cause less sleep disturbance and nightmares. Water-soluble beta blockers are excreted by the kidneys and dosage reduction is often necessary in renal impairment. Nightmares and sleep disturbance is a common adverse effect of propranolol according to the SmPC. Acronym for water soluble beta-blockers: SNAC – sotalol, nadolol, atenolol & celiprolol.
https://bnf.nice.org.uk/treatment-summaries/beta-adrenoceptor-blocking-drugs/

43 **A - Amlodipine**
Contraindications of amlodipine are cardiogenic shock, significant aortic stenosis and unstable angina.

Additional information:
- Ramipril: max. daily dose 5 mg if creatinine clearance 30–60 ml/min.
- Orbit score of 0-2 = low risk of bleeding
- DOACs may not be appropriate in patients with a BMI > 40 kg/m2 or a weight > 120kg due to the risk of under-dosing.
- Apixaban should be reduced to 2.5 mg BD if serum-creatinine ≥133 micromol/L PLUS ≥80 years old OR ≤60 kg (also reduce dose to 2.5 mg BD if CrCl 15–29 ml/min).

https://bnf.nice.org.uk/drug/amlodipine.html?msclkid=b62360f5a9e411 ec8406a7a743b254ed

44   E - Dipyridamole 200mg modified-release capsules plus aspirin 75mg tablets

The standard treatment is clopidogrel 75mg daily. If clopidogrel cannot be tolerated, aspirin 75mg daily plus MR dipyridamole 200mg BD. If both clopidogrel & aspirin are contraindicated or cannot be tolerated: MR dipyridamole 200mg twice daily alone. If both clopidogrel & MR dipyridamole are contraindicated or cannot be tolerated: Aspirin 75mg daily alone may be used. Treatment with a high-intensity statin (such as atorvastatin 20–80 mg daily) will be offered at diagnosis of ischaemic stroke or TIA by secondary care.

https://cks.nice.org.uk/topics/stroke-tia/management/suspected-transient-ischaemic-attack/

45   E - Preparation

The patient is aware of the problem and plans to make the change away from their harmful behaviour. Additional information:
- Pre-contemplation: no intention of changing behaviour
- Contemplation: the individual is aware of the inherent risks of their actions and is weighing up the pros and cons
- Preparation: the patient is intending to take action to address the problem
- Action: the individual has made the move to alter their harmful behaviour
- Maintenance: the individual has not engaged in their harmful behaviour

Nitrous oxide is covered by the Psychoactive Substances Act and is illegal to supply for its psychoactive effect.

https://exploringyourmind.com/prochaska-diclementes-transtheoretical-model-of-change/

46 D - Ondansetron

Metoclopramide is recommended to be used for up to 5 days and is not known to be harmful in pregnancy. Ondansetron is recommended to be used for up to 5 days. Manufacturer advises to avoid in the first trimester due to a small increased risk of congenital abnormalities such as orofacial clefts.

Additional information:

Domperidone should not be prescribed for longer than 7 days.

https://cks.nice.org.uk/topics/nausea-vomiting-in-pregnancy/ management/management/

47 C - Lithium

Lithium should be stopped 24 hours before major surgery, however in a minor surgery the usual dose can be continued with careful monitoring.

Additional Information:

Drugs that should be stopped before surgery:

Hormone contraceptives, MAOIs, ACEI/ARBS (stop 24 hours before surgery). Lithium should be stopped 24 hours before major surgery, however in a minor surgery the usual dose can be continued with careful monitoring

Drugs that should NOT be stopped before surgery:

Antiepileptics, antiparkinsonian drugs, antipsychotics, anxiolytics, bronchodilators, cardiovascular drugs, glaucoma drugs, immuno-suppressants, drugs of dependence, and thyroid or antithyroid drugs.

https://bnf.nice.org.uk/treatment-summary/surgery-and-long-term-medication.html

48 C - 5–7mmol/L

The optimal targets for glucose self-monitoring in adults with type 1 diabetes are:

- Fasting plasma glucose level of 5–7mmol/L on waking
- Plasma glucose level of 4–7mmol/L before meals at other times of the day
- For adults who choose to test after meals, plasma glucose level of 5–9mmol/L at least 90 minutes after eating

https://cks.nice.org.uk/topics/diabetes-type-1/management/management-adults/

49 **C - Refer to GP urgently**

Patients taking carbimazole should always be warned about the onset of sore throats, bruising or bleeding, mouth ulcers, fever and malaise and should be instructed to stop the drug and to seek medical advice immediately. In such patients, white blood cell counts should be performed immediately, particularly where there is any clinical evidence of infection. This can be done in a GP surgery without having to go to A&E.

Additional information:

Carbimazole should be stopped promptly if there is clinical or laboratory evidence of neutropenia.

https://bnf.nice.org.uk/drug/carbimazole.html

50 **D - Linagliptin**

The patient is currently at the first intensification of the diabetic management. The next option would be to add in a second antidiabetic mediation or insulin. See below for the rationale:

- Canagliflozin is inappropriate due to the MHRA/CHM advice: SGLT2 inhibitors: reports of Fournier's gangrene (necrotising fasciitis of the genitalia or perineum). Fournier's gangrene, a rare but serious and potentially life-threatening infection, has been associated with the use of sodium-glucose co-transporter 2 (SGLT2) inhibitors.
- Glimepiride: the patient is already taking a sulfonylurea, therefore it is inappropriate to add this to the regime.
- Exenatide (GLP-1 mimetic): whilst GLP-1 mimetics can improve blood glucose control, it requires the use of injections. However, the patient has phobia of needles and patient preference should be taken into consideration when starting any new medicine.
- Pioglitazone is contraindicated in patients with a history of heart failure, previous or active bladder cancer and uninvestigated macroscopic haematuria.
- Linagliptin would be the safest option in view of the patient past medical history and preference.

https://cks.nice.org.uk/diabetes-type-2#!scenario
https://bnf.nice.org.uk/treatment-summary/type-2-diabetes.html

51 **B - Cefalexin 500mg BD for 7 days**

Nitrofurantoin is usually first choice but should be prescribed for 7 days in pregnancy. Amoxicillin & pivmecillinam would be inappropriate due to penicillin allergy. Trimethoprim manufacturers advise to avoid during pregnancy, particularly in the first trimester due to the risk of teratogenicity. Cefalexin is safe to use in pregnancy and a duration of 7 days is appropriate for pregnant women.

Additional information:

Nitrofurantoin should be avoided at term (36-42 weeks).

https://bnf.nice.org.uk/treatment-summary/urinary-tract-infections.html

52 D - Flucloxacillin

Important safety information: Cholestatic jaundice and hepatitis may occur, very rarely, up to two months after treatment with flucloxacillin has been stopped. Administration for more than 2 weeks and increasing age are risk factors.

https://bnf.nice.org.uk/drug/flucloxacillin.html#importantSafetyInformations

53 C - Chloramphenicol IV

For the treatment of meningococcal diseases, benzylpenicillin is recommended or cefotaxime if allergic to penicillin. If there is a history of immediate hypersensitivity reaction (including anaphylaxis, angioedema, urticaria, or rash immediately after administration) to penicillin or to cephalosporins, chloramphenicol can be used. Tigecycline (tetracycline antibiotic) is contraindicated in children under the age of 8 years old due to the risk of deposition in growing bones and teeth. Teicoplanin should not be given by mouth for systemic infections because it is not absorbed significantly. It is also not indicated to treat meningitis.

Additional information:

The treatment of meningococcal diseases can be found towards the back of the BNF (shiny pages) - Medical emergencies in the community.

https://bnf.nice.org.uk/treatment-summary/medical-emergencies-in-the-community.html?msclkid=ab04bbceaae511eca666af2cdd80c999

54 A – Apixaban

Reduce dose if serum creatinine $\geq$ 1.5 mg/dL (133 micromole/L)

https://bnf.nice.org.uk/drugs/apixaban/#renalImpairment

55 **E – Warfarin**
This is usually indicated for patients with heart valves and the DOACS are usually indicated for non valvular patients.
https://bnf.nice.org.uk/drugs/warfarin-sodium/#indicationsAndDoses

56 **C – Clopidogrel**
This is due to an interaction risk (see alert below)
https://www.gov.uk/drug-safety-update/clopidogrel-and-proton-pump-inhibitors-interaction-updated-advice?msclkid=56812194cf1911ec8dff9469d4ab78ad

57 **D – Dipyridamole**
The frequency is not known but it can cause hypotension.
https://bnf.nice.org.uk/drugs/dipyridamole/#sideEffects

58 **A – Apixaban**
As per manufacturers guidance, this can help support compliance.
https://www.medicines.org.uk/emc/product/13686/smpc

59 **A - ACE inhibitor**
This is the first line recommended drug.
https://www.nice.org.uk/guidance/NG136?msclkid=f66d7db2cf1911ec86e042e8243e207d

60 **D - Blood pressure, renal function and electrolytes (recommended monitoring)**
https://bnf.nice.org.uk/treatment-summaries/drugs-affecting-the-renin-angiotensin-system/

61 **A - Concomitant drug therapy with another NSAID**
This is due to the risk of bleed.
https://cks.nice.org.uk/topics/nsaids-prescribing-issues/

62 **E - Refer him to his GP with a note suggesting prescribing naproxen plus lansoprazole 15mg daily**
Avoid ibuprofen. There are no urgent red flags listed so refer to a GP with an appropriate suggestion.

ANSWERS

63   **E - Oral morphine M/R tablets 50mg bd**
Codeine 30mg 2 qds = Codeine 240mg = Morphine salt 24mg daily
Buprenorphine 20mcg patch = Morphine salt 48mg daily
Oramorph 2.5ml qds = Morphine salt 20mg daily
Total morphine salt daily = 92mg daily
Need to provide a dose which is a little higher than current dose as pain is
uncontrolled. Fentanyl 50 patch would be too high a jump. IV morphine
inappropriate at this stage of therapy.
https://bnf.nice.org.uk/guidance/prescribing-in-palliative-care.html

64   **D - Triggers may include dehydration, irregular meals, tiredness, and
stress.**
For most patients who suffer with migraines, there are often trigger
factors which can cause the migraine to occur.
https://bnf.nice.org.uk/treatment-summary/migraine.html

65   **C – Crifampicin**
This is an enzyme inducer.
*https://nursingnotes.co.uk/resources/cytochrome-p450-inducers-inhibitors-
mnemonic/#.Ynl3kOjMK3A*

66   **E - Sodium valproate**
This is an enzyme inhibitor.
*https://nursingnotes.co.uk/resources/cytochrome-p450-inducers-inhibitors-
mnemonic/#.Ynl3kOjMK3A*

67   **A – Aminophylline**
There is an interaction, thus increasing the risk of digoxin toxicity.
https://bnf.nice.org.uk/interaction/digoxin-2.html#bnf_i1649038987697

68   **B - Awareness of hypoglycaemia signs and symptoms and how to manage
these should be assessed and reinforced at annual reviews with patients**
See further reading on how to manage these events.
https://bnf.nice.org.uk/treatment-summaries/hypoglycaemia/

69   **C - Neuropathic pain can respond to opioids**
The pain can respond well to opioids if prescribed appropriately.
https://bnf.nice.org.uk/treatment-summaries/neuropathic-pain/

70 D - You should ensure Mrs FS has an appointment for her next annual blood test and advise to return if she experiences signs or symptoms of hypothyroidism
All parameters are in range so it is safe to continue at the current dose.
https://cks.nice.org.uk/topics/hypothyroidism/

71 C - Glimepiride
Sulfonylureas can cause weight gain.
https://bnf.nice.org.uk/treatment-summary/type-2-diabetes.html

72 G - Pioglitazone
This is due to bladder cancer risk.
https://bnf.nice.org.uk/drug/pioglitazone.html

73 H - Repaglinide
As per manufacturers license for indication.
https://bnf.nice.org.uk/treatment-summary/type-2-diabetes.html

74 D - Nitrofurantoin
Safe to issue in pregnancy.
https://bnf.nice.org.uk/treatment-summaries/urinary-tract-infections/

75 C - Flucloxacillin
Usually first line in cellulitis.
https://cks.nice.org.uk/topics/cellulitis-acute/?msclkid=475eb01dcf1d11ec9 0eb08ca1b45c99c

76 H - None of the above
https://cks.nice.org.uk/topics/fungal-nail-infection/?msclkid=5d2a7ba9cf1 d11ec8727e78301127d16

77 H - None of the above
https://cks.nice.org.uk/topics/chest-infections-adult/management/acute-br onchitis/?msclkid=7c3e263ccf1d11ecaade21d45d453aa3

78 C - Lansoprazole 30mg bd, clarithromycin 500mg bd, metronidazole 400mg bd
Options A, B, and D contain penicillin antibiotic. Option E contains omeprazole which interacts with clopidogrel.
https://bnf.nice.org.uk/treatment-summaries/helicobacter-pylori-infection/

ANSWERS

79 **D - Presence should be confirmed before starting eradication therapy.**
It should ideally be confirmed before initiation.
https://bnf.nice.org.uk/treatment-summaries/helicobacter-pylori-infection/

80 **A - Request a sputum sample for culture and susceptibility**
This will help issue the correct antibiotic.
*https://cks.nice.org.uk/topics/chronic-obstructive-pulmonary-disease/
management/acute-exacerbation/*

81 **B - Ramipril, bisoprolol, aspirin, clopidogrel and atorvastatin**
These are all prescribed as secondary prevention.
https://cks.nice.org.uk/topics/mi-secondary-prevention/

82 **D - This is a sign of severe acute asthma and patient needs referral to A&E**
This is due to the severe symptoms.
https://bnf.nice.org.uk/treatment-summaries/asthma-acute/

83 **E - No prescription needed due to likely viral indication**
The patient's observations are all okay, the patient can be safety netted for
worsening symptoms.

84 **A - Check inhaler technique and add montelukast 10mg OD**
As per asthma stepwise therapy.
https://bnf.nice.org.uk/treatment-summaries/asthma-chronic/

85 **A - Decrease dose of uniphyllin continus after checking levels (stopping
smoking)**
Smoking can increase theophylline clearance and increased doses of
theophylline are therefore required; dose adjustments are likely to be
necessary if smoking started or stopped during treatment.
https://bnf.nice.org.uk/drugs/theophylline/

86 **C - 10-20mg/Litre**
https://bnf.nice.org.uk/drugs/aminophylline/

87 **B - Full blood count and renal and liver function tests every 3 months**
Patient has now been stabilised on this medication by his consultant
therefore the long term monitoring is now needed.
https://bnf.nice.org.uk/drugs/methotrexate/#monitoringRequirements

88 **A - Chest x-ray, potassium levels, liver function tests, and thyroid function tests**
https://bnf.nice.org.uk/drugs/amiodarone-hydrochloride/

89 **A - Allopurinol**
This prevents hyperuricaemia.
https://bnf.nice.org.uk/drugs/allopurinol/#indications-and-dose

90 **A - 100mg of phenytoin sodium is approximately equivalent to 92mg phenytoin base**
https://bnf.nice.org.uk/drugs/phenytoin/

91 **B - 15mg once daily**
This is the correct dose according to the patient parameters.
https://www.medicines.org.uk/emc/product/2793/smpch
https://bnf.nice.org.uk/guidance/prescribing-in-renal-impairment.html

92 **A - For plasma digoxin levels, bloods should be taken 6 hours after the dose**
This is the correct monitoring of plasma levels.
https://bnf.nice.org.uk/drugs/digoxin/

93 **A - Avoid NSAID's in this patient due to risk factors**
Avoid due to cardiovascular risk factors. If the patient were to be initiated on NSAID therapy then they would need a clinical review with a prescriber to discuss risks versus benefits. Ibuprofen can be prescribed if appropriate. The statement states 'avoid' so try to do this if possible. His last BP reading was also raised.
https://cks.nice.org.uk/topics/nsaids-prescribing-issues/

94 **B - Report any symptoms of diabetic ketoacidosis**
There is an MHRA alert regarding the risk of diabetic ketoacidosis, patients should be counselled when treatment is initiated.
https://bnf.nice.org.uk/drugs/dapagliflozin/

95 **C - Omit warfarin for 2 days then return to 3mg OD dose**
Mr BC has been on holiday and returned back to his normal lifestyle/diet

ANSWERS

so the INR should correct itself. As the INR is raised and warfarin has a half life of 72 hours, omitting the dose for 2 days will help levels to correct themselves. Stopping warfarin for 1-2 weeks is dangerous; there is also no need for an A&E admission (no bleeding).
https://bnf.nice.org.uk/drugs/warfarin-sodium/

96 B - Course of antibiotics, e.g. flucloxacillin as this is potentially an infected boil and also hot, compression on the area
Advising mum regarding hot compression is good advice but the patient is in pain and has a temperature, therefore antibiotics in addition will be needed.
https://cks.nice.org.uk/topics/boils-carbuncles-staphylococcal-carriage/ diagnosis/clinical-presentation-of-a-boil/

97 D - Advise the GP to recommend an alternative to tramadol
Alternative needed if possible (there is a risk of serotonin syndrome, interaction between tramadol and fluoxetine).
https://www.medicines.org.uk/emc/product/7123/smpc

98 B - Dihydrocodeine can be used during labour in pregnancy
It can be used for moderate to severe pain.
https://bnf.nice.org.uk/drugs/dihydrocodeine-tartrate/#indications-and-dose

99 D - Remind patient of risks, not to try to conceive until discussing with specialist
Teratogenic risks with valproate and pregnancy – the patient is not to try to conceive and should have signed a pregnancy prevention programme. The patient needs to discuss her plans with her specialist so her medication can be changed.
https://bnf.nice.org.uk/drugs/sodium-valproate/

100 A - Folic acid 5mg to be taken once daily (apart from Wednesdays)
This is the only appropriate/safe dose listed alongside methotrexate therapy.
https://bnf.nice.org.uk/drugs/folic-acid/

Medium weighted answers

101 **E - Take urlipristal 30mg stat**
Urlipristal is effective if taken within 120 hours (5 days) of unprotected intercourse, since the patient described it as just under 5 days, urlipristal is the most appropriate. Copper IUD is the most effective however due to timespan, there may be a delay in obtaining device.
https://bnf.nice.org.uk/treatment-summaries/emergency-contraception/

102 **C - Metronidazole 0.75% vaginal gel – use nightly for 5 nights**
During lactation, metronidazole enters breast milk and can alter the taste of breast milk, therefore avoid oral treatment in lactating women and use topical treatment instead. Clindamycin vaginal cream can be used but it is expensive. Clotrimazole is used for candidiasis not bacterial vaginosis so would not be effective.
https://cks.nice.org.uk/topics/bacterial-vaginosis/

103 **B - BP 163/101**
This would represent an unacceptable health risk if the method is used. Consult literature by the faculty of sexual & reproductive healthcare – UKMEC summary table for more information.
https://www.fsrh.org/site-search/?keywords=ukmec+summary

104 **B - Levonogestrel–releasing intrauterine device**
The rest interact with phenytoin since it is an enzyme inducing drug and there are known clinical interactions. See FSRH CEU guidelines – drug interactions with hormonal contraception.
https://www.fsrh.org/standards-and-guidance/documents/ceu-clinical-guidance-drug-interactions-with-hormonal/

ANSWERS

105 **D - Oral phosphodiesterase type-5 inhibitor is the first line drug treatment and acts by initiating an erection**

Oral phosphodiesterase type-5 inhibitor is the first line drug treatment and acts by initiating an erection. Oral phosphodiesterase type-5 inhibitor is indeed the first line drug treatment however it acts by increasing blood flow to the penis – it is sexual stimulation that initiates an erection and not the tablet itself.

https://bnf.nice.org.uk/treatment-summaries/erectile-dysfunction/

106 **E - Hypomagnesaemia**

The MHRA have warned of the risk of hypomagnesaemia following prolonged use of PPIs (>1 year). Serious manifestations of hypomagnesaemia include fatigue, tetany, delirium, convulsions, dizziness, and ventricular arrhythmia. For patients expected to be on prolonged treatment, and especially for those who take PPIs with digoxin or drugs that may cause hypomagnesaemia (e.g., diuretics), healthcare professionals should consider measuring magnesium levels before starting PPI treatment and repeat measurements periodically during treatment.

https://www.gov.uk/drug-safety-update/proton-pump-inhibitors-in-long-term-use-reports-of-hypomagnesaemia

107 **C - Ispaghula husk**

Ispaghula husk is a bulk forming laxative and these have been advised to be avoided in opioid-induced constipation.

https://bnf.nice.org.uk/drug/ispaghula-husk.html

108 **E – Vomiting**

All other options are typical symptoms.

https://cks.nice.org.uk/topics/irritable-bowel-syndrome/

109 **A - A patient with a BMI of 26 who is diagnosed with type 2 diabetes**

Orlistat - adjunct in obesity (in conjunction with a mildly hypocaloric diet in individuals with a body mass index (BMI) of 30kg/m2 or more or in individuals with a BMI of 28kg/m2 or more in the presence of other risk factors such as type 2 diabetes, hypertension, or hypercholesterolaemia).

https://bnf.nice.org.uk/drug/orlistat.html

110 **A - Antibiotics are not recommended for patients with diverticular disease**
As per the recommendations.
https://cks.nice.org.uk/topics/diverticular-disease/management/

111 **D - Hypokalaemia**
Plasma potassium concentration may be reduced by beta-2 agonists (particularly high doses). Plasma potassium should be monitored in severe asthma.

112 **B - Add in relvar ellipta 92/22 micrograms inhaler**
ICS/LABA since patients FEV1<50. The patient was hospitalised a week ago and eosinophils are raised, therefore most appropriate treatment is to use ICS/LABA.
https://cks.nice.org.uk/topics/chronic-obstructive-pulmonary-disease/

113 **E - Simvastatin**
There is an increased risk of myopathy (due to cytochrome P450 enzyme CYP3A4 inhibition). For simvastatin (potent CYP3A4 inhibitor), concurrent use is contraindicated. If clarithromycin treatment cannot be avoided, stop treatment with simvastatin during the course of the treatment.
https://bnf.nice.org.uk/interactions/simvastatin/

114 **B - 10 – 20mg/L**
In most individuals, a plasma-theophylline concentration of 10–20mg/litre (55–110 micromol/litre) is required for satisfactory bronchodilation, although a lower plasma-theophylline concentration of 5–15mg/litre may be effective.
https://bnf.nice.org.uk/drugs/aminophylline/

115 **E - Raised PaCO2 and/or the need for mechanical ventilation with raised inflation pressures This is due to raised carbon monoxide.**
https://bnf.nice.org.uk/treatment-summary/asthma-acute.html

116 **D - Megaloblastic anaemia**
Most megaloblastic anaemias result from a lack of either vitamin B12 or folate.
https://cks.nice.org.uk/topics/anaemia-b12-folate-deficiency/

ANSWERS

	Electrolyte imbalance	Treatment
117	**Hyperkalaemia**	Calcium resonium®
118	Hyponatraemia	**Slow Sodium®**
119	**Hypocalcaemia**	Sandocal 1000® effervescent tablets
120	**Hypophosphataemia**	Phosphate sandoz® effervescent tablet

117 Hyperkalaemia

Calcium resonium exchanges potassium in the blood for calcium, therefore reducing the amount of potassium in the blood.
https://bnf.nice.org.uk/treatment-summaries/fluids-and-electrolytes/

118 Slow Sodium

Slow sodium is used for hyponatraemia, this is where the amount of sodium in the body is low.
https://cks.nice.org.uk/topics/hyponatraemia/

119 Hypocalcaemia

Sandocal 1000 effervescent tablets; for mild cases of hypocalcaemia where there is less calcium in the body. Note: magnesium levels should be checked as hypomagnesaemia can cause secondary hypocalcaemia.
https://bnf.nice.org.uk/drugs/calcium-carbonate-with-calcium-lactate-gluconate/#prescribing-and-dispensing-information

120 Hypophosphataemia

Phosphate Sandoz effervescent tablet, for mild deficiency of phosphate oral therapy is safer and should be used wherever possible.
https://bnf.nice.org.uk/drugs/phosphate/#indications-and-dose

121 A - No, she does not need contraception

She is >55years old and the chance of spontaneous conception at this age is extremely rare.
https://cks.nice.org.uk/topics/pre-conception-advice-management/

122 A - Blood pressure.

See MHRA risk regarding raised blood pressure.
https://www.gov.uk/drug-safety-update/mirabegron-betmiga-risk-of-severe-hypertension-and-associated-cerebrovascular-and-cardiac-events
https://bnf.nice.org.uk/drug/mirabegron.html

123 **C - Rectal examination and PSA blood test**

Blood in the urine is a red flag symptom that needs further investigation. It can sometimes be present as part of a urine infection of which he had symptoms, e.g. urgency/frequency. However, this patient's sample came back normal and because he is in the 'at-risk age group' for prostate cancer, the next steps would involve a rectal examination and PSA test. The results from these determine the urgency of a referral to urology if at all, if for example, PSA is raised or the examination shows an enlarged/changed prostate.

https://cks.nice.org.uk/topics/prostate-cancer/

124 **E - Vitamin B12 deficiency**

PPIs inhibit the production of gastric acid which is needed to aid the absorption of vitamin B12. Thus, medicines that interfere with gastric acid can contribute to/enhance a vitamin B12 deficiency.

https://www.medicines.org.uk/emc/product/5944/smpc

125 **D - Inflammation and continuous partial thickness in the rectum that extends through the colon**

Description as per NICE guidelines for UC, 'occurs in rectum but extends a variable distance through colon'. With Crohn's, it can occur anywhere between the mouth and anus and the inflammation is not continuous but there is full thickness.

https://cks.nice.org.uk/topics/ulcerative-colitis/

126 **B - Shake the inhaler, take the cap off and breathe out gently to empty the lungs. Put your lips around the mouthpiece, start to breathe in slowly and steadily and at the same time press the cannister down once. Continue to breathe in slowly until your lungs feel full, then hold for 10 seconds, or as long as comfortable, and leave at least 30 seconds between a second dose**

Technique for MDI as per Asthma UK. Important points to remember for MDI's is the importance of coordinating actuation and inhalation and that breathing must be slow and steady.

https://www.asthma.org.uk/

127 D - Height and weight annually

This is part of the monitoring that is needed for children.
*https://bnf.nice.org.uk/drug/beclometasone-dipropionate.
html#indicationsAndDoses*

128 E – Thiamine

This is used for the prevention of encephalopathy.
https://bnf.nice.org.uk/drug/thiamine.html

129 A - Although best absorbed on an empty stomach, advise to take after food to reduce gastro-intestinal side effects

Taken after food to prevent GI related symptoms such as change in bowels.
https://bnf.nice.org.uk/drugs/ferrous-sulfate/#indications-and-dose

130 C - One or two 50mg tablets should be taken with water approximately one hour before anticipated sexual activity

The maximum dose of Viagra connect is ONE 50mg tablet per day (P). For the POM product only: based on efficacy and tolerability, the dose may be increased to 100mg or decreased to 25mg. The maximum recommended dose is 100mg.

Hint: The other options listed are correct statements and can be used to supplement knowledge.
https://www.rpharMscom/resources/quick-reference-guides/sildenafil-50mg-film-coated-tablets-p-medicine

131 B - Intrauterine copper device

From the list, ulipristal 30mg, levonorgestrel 1500 microgram and copper intrauterine device are the only options for emergency contraception. Women requiring emergency contraception who are using enzyme-inducing drugs should be offered a Copper-IUD if appropriate. Limited data from clinical trials suggest a possible trend for a reduced contraceptive efficacy of ulipristal acetate with high body weight or BMI. Similar trends are seen with LNG. Although a double dose of LNG can be given, this is not advisable first line.
https://www.fsrh.org/standards-and-guidance/fsrh-guidelines-and-statements/emergency-contraception/

132 D - Levonorgestrel 150 microgram/ethinylestradiol 30 microgram tablets

Levonorgestrel/ethinylestradiol is a combined hormonal contraceptive which increases the risk of thrombosis in patients undergoing major surgery and should be discontinued at least 4 weeks prior to major surgery. Progestogen-only pills, injections, implants, and intra-uterine systems are suitable for use as contraceptives in females undergoing surgery.

Additional information:

Combined hormone contraceptive may be recommenced 2 weeks after full remobilisation.

https://bnf.nice.org.uk/treatment-summary/contraceptives-hormonal.html

133 C - Refer to GP urgently

Sulfasalazine can cause blood disorders. Patients receiving aminosalicylates, and their carers, should be advised to report any unexplained bleeding, bruising, purpura, sore throat, fever, or malaise that occurs during treatment.

Additional Information:

Purpura - a rash of purple spots on the skin caused by internal bleeding from small blood vessels.

https://bnf.nice.org.uk/drug/sulfasalazine.
html?msclkid=1374b64fabba11ec8fdeeab318e0d2cf

134 B - Co-danthrusate

Co-danthramer & co-danthrusate is indicated for constipation in palliative care. Rodent studies indicate potential carcinogenic risk. An adverse effect is that it can change the colour of urine to red.

https://bnf.nice.org.uk/drug/co-danthramer.html

135 G - Senna

Senna has an onset of action 8–12 hours and can discolour urine. Bisacodyl: tablets act in 10–12 hours, suppositories work in 20–60 minutes. Docusate: oral preparations act within 1–2 days, suppositories work in 20 minutes. Bulk forming laxative: onset of action 72 hours.

Additional information:

Senna available for general sale has been limited to a pack size of two short treatment courses (up to 20 standard-strength tablets, 10 maximum-

strength tablets or 100ml solution/syrup). MHRA/CHM advice: stimulant laxatives (bisacodyl, senna and sennosides, sodium picosulfate) available over-the-counter: new measures to support safe use.
https://bnf.nice.org.uk/drug/senna.
html?msclkid=86792eeeac0511ec9151cc521759cc8f

136 A - 150mcg, then repeated after 5–15 minutes as required

For a child 1 month–5 years (<15kg): 150mcg. For a child 6–11 years (>30kg): 300mcg. For a child 12 years old and over: 500mcg
https://bnfc.nice.org.uk/drug/adrenalineepinephrine.html

137 B - Heart failure

Factors that decrease theophylline concentration: smoking, alcohol, St John's wort, rifampicin (this list is not exhaustive).
Factors that increase theophylline concentration: heart failure, hepatic impairment and viral infections.
https://bnf.nice.org.uk/drug/theophylline.html#interactions

138 D - Luforbec (formoterol + beclometasone)

MART is only available for inhaled corticosteroid (ICS) and long acting B2 agonist (LABA) combinations where the B2 agonist is fast-acting, e.g. formoterol. Although salmeterol is a long acting B2 agonist, it has a slower onset of action therefore unsuitable for MART regimes.
https://bnf.nice.org.uk/treatment-summary/asthma-chronic.html

139 E - Vitamin B12

Vitamin B12 is combined with a protein called intrinsic factor in the stomach, this then allows the vitamin B12 complex to be absorbed into the body.
Additional information:
Drugs reducing vitamin B12: colchicine, metformin, nitrous oxide, protein pump inhibitors, H2-receptor antagonists.
https://cks.nice.org.uk/topics/anaemia-b12-folate-deficiency/background-information/causes/#pernicious-anaemia

140 F - Vitamin C

This is the treatment for scurvy.

https://bnf.nice.org.uk/treatment-summary/vitamins.html

141 A - Vitamin A

It should be avoided in pregnancy.

https://bnf.nice.org.uk/treatment-summary/vitamins.html

142 G - Vitamin D

There is a higher risk of deficiency in darker skin tones.

https://bnf.nice.org.uk/treatment-summary/vitamins.html

143 H - Vitamin K

A reversal agent for warfarin.

https://bnf.nice.org.uk/treatment-summary/vitamins.html

144 H - Hypomagnesaemia

Proton pump inhibitors (PPI's) are known to decrease magnesium levels (usually after one year of treatment).

Additional information:

PPI's can also increase the risk of osteoporosis. Hypomagnesaemia in very low levels can present with muscle weakness and tremors, seizures, and irregular heart rhythms

https://bnf.nice.org.uk/drug/lansoprazole.
html?msclkid=16d0ed98ac1d11ec9a760bbfe2d4395f

145 G - Hyponatraemia

Hyponatraemia (usually in the elderly and possibly due to inappropriate secretion of antidiuretic hormone) has been associated with all types of antidepressants; however, it has been reported more frequently with SSRIs than with other antidepressants.

https://bnf.nice.org.uk/treatment-summary/antidepressant-drugs.html

146 A - Hypercalcaemia

The drug is indicated for hypercalcaemia in malignancy.

https://bnf.nice.org.uk/drug/pamidronate-disodium.
html#indicationsAndDoses

ANSWERS

147 F - Hypoglycaemia

In diabetes mellitus patients with frequent hypoglycaemic episodes (risk of suppressing hypoglycaemic symptoms).
https://bnf.nice.org.uk/drug/bisoprolol-fumarate.html

148 C – Hyperkalaemia

Due to combination of diuretic with spironolactone.
https://bnf.nice.org.uk/drug/spironolactone.html#sideEffects

149 A - Bleomycin

All cytotoxic cause bone marrow suppression except for vincristine and bleomycin.
https://bnf.nice.org.uk/treatment-summary/cytotoxic-drugs.html

150 D – Doxorubicin

As per BNF information re product formulation.
https://bnf.nice.org.uk/drug/doxorubicin-hydrochloride.html

151 H – Vinblastine

Never administer intrathecally.
https://bnf.nice.org.uk/drug/vincristine-sulfate.html

152 F – Methotrexate

Needs regular routine monitoring when issued to patients.
https://bnf.nice.org.uk/drug/methotrexate.html

153 B - Methotrexate

Azathioprine: contraceptive precautions should be advised whilst either partner is receiving azathioprine. Mycophenolate: Male patients or their female partner should use effective contraception during treatment and for 90 days after discontinuation. Sulfasalazine: patients should be advised to use contraception during treatment. Tacrolimus: advised to use a reliable means of contraception during and for at least three months after treatment.
https://bnf.nice.org.uk/treatment-summary/cytotoxic-drugs.html?msclkid=dc56ed23ac2111ecac69bd6cf89104e7

154 **E - Piroxicam**
GI risk: (high) piroxicam, ketoprofen, ketorolac → (intermediate) indometacin, diclofenac, naproxen →(low) ibuprofen 1.2g/day → (lowest) COX-2 selective inhibitors.
https://bnf.nice.org.uk/treatment-summary/non-steroidal-anti-inflammatory-drugs.html?msclkid=65f59ff7ac2c11ec9ca00d5423bd7068

155 **E - All of the above.**
Sildenafil can be prescribed and/or issued in the community safely as long as contra-indications and cautions are considered.
https://bnf.nice.org.uk/drug/sildenafil.html
https://cks.nice.org.uk/topics/cvd-risk-assessment-management/
https://www.nhs.uk/live-well/healthy-weight/bmi-calculator/

156 **C - Mrs TW should be advised to explore alternative contraceptive methods**
She requires a more potent contraceptive method.
https://www.fsrh.org/standards-and-guidance/documents/ceu-clinical-guidance-drug-interactions-with-hormonal/

157 **D - Taking a CHC with no hormone-free interval is a licenced regimen, useful for patients with heavy or painful withdrawal bleeds**
It is not licensed.
https://bnf.nice.org.uk/treatment-summary/contraceptives-hormonal.html
https://bnf.nice.org.uk/treatment-summary/sex-hormones.html
https://bnf.nice.org.uk/drug/desogestrel.html
https://www.fsrh.org/standards-and-guidance/documents/ceu-clinical-guidance-drug-interactions-with-hormonal/
https://bnf.nice.org.uk/drug/clonidine-hydrochloride.html

158 **B - Prescribe intravaginal metronidazole gel 0.75% once daily for 5 days.**
Oral may not be appropriate due to alcohol reference from patient.
https://cks.nice.org.uk/topics/bacterial-vaginosis/

159 **B - Miss GR should start taking her Cerelle tablets immediately**
Females should wait 5 days after taking ulipristal acetate before starting suitable hormonal contraception.
https://bnf.nice.org.uk/treatment-summary/emergency-contraception.html

160 E - None of the above

https://bnf.nice.org.uk/treatment-summary/helicobacter-pylori-infection.html
https://bnf.nice.org.uk/treatment-summary/dyspepsia.html
https://cks.nice.org.uk/topics/dyspepsia-unidentified-cause/

161 C – Diarrhoea

A symptom associated with Crohn's.
https://bnf.nice.org.uk/drug/colestyramine.html

162 C – Diarrhoea

A recent course of antibiotics or long term use of PPI can cause this to occur.
https://cks.nice.org.uk/topics/diarrhoea-antibiotic-associated/
management/diarrhoea-antibiotic-associated/

163 E - All of the above

All the symptoms listed are potential side effects.
https://bnf.nice.org.uk/drug/ferrous-fumarate.html

164 B – Constipation

As per licensing when other treatment options have failed.
https://bnf.nice.org.uk/drug/prucalopride.html

165 E - All of the above

https://cks.nice.org.uk/topics/gastrointestinal-tract-upper-cancers-recognition-referral/background-information/presentation/

166 C - Check inhaler technique

https://cks.nice.org.uk/topics/asthma/management/follow-up/

167 E - Suggest that Mrs LR could reduce her Fostair to 1 puff bd

Can step down patient due to stable symptoms.
https://www.nice.org.uk/guidance/ng80
https://www.nice.org.uk/guidance/ng80/chapter/
Recommendations#decreasing-maintenance-therapy

168 E - This patient is not indicated for pneumococcal vaccine

https://bnf.nice.org.uk/treatment-summary/chronic-obstructive-pulmonary-disease.html

169 **E - None of the above**
https://bnf.nice.org.uk/treatment-summary/chronic-obstructive-pulmonary-disease.html
https://bnf.nice.org.uk/treatment-summary/respiratory-system-drug-delivery.html
https://bnf.nice.org.uk/drug/roflumilast.html
https://bnf.nice.org.uk/drug/azithromycin.html

170 **D - Requires warning label 2 to be added to dispensing labels**
This is listed in the BNF.
https://bnf.nice.org.uk/drug/fexofenadine-hydrochloride.html
https://bnf.nice.org.uk/about/labels.html

171 **E - Hydroxocobalamin I/M; initially 1mg 3 times a week for 2 weeks, then 1mg every 3 months**
This is a usual dose for this type of anaemia.
https://cks.nice.org.uk/topics/anaemia-b12-folate-deficiency/

172 **C - Folic acid 5mg weekly, on a different day to the methotrexate dose**
https://bnf.nice.org.uk/drug/folic-acid.html

173 **D - 5mg daily started before conception until week 12 of pregnancy**
https://bnf.nice.org.uk/drug/folic-acid.html

174 **D - Support the breast-feeding parent to eliminate all cow's milk from their diet and prescribe calcium and vitamin D supplementation**
https://cks.nice.org.uk/topics/cows-milk-allergy-in-children/management/suspected-cows-milk-allergy/

175 **D - Stop treatment and contact specialty department for advice**
Due to the abnormal blood results whilst taking DMARD.
https://cks.nice.org.uk/topics/dmards/

ANSWERS

Low weighted answers

176 F – Tamoxifen

This is usually prescribed for five years for prevention.

https://bnf.nice.org.uk/drugs/tamoxifen/

177 D – Methotrexate

This is usually an option for this indication (azathioprine can be trialled if methotrexate failed to work for the patient).

https://bnf.nice.org.uk/drugs/methotrexate/
https://bnf.nice.org.uk/drugs/azathioprine/#indications-and-dose

178 B – Bicalutamide

Can be used with an analogue for prostate cancer.

https://bnf.nice.org.uk/drugs/bicalutamide/

179 E – Tacrolimus

A calcineurin inhibitor which is usually prescribed to prevent graft rejection.

https://bnf.nice.org.uk/drugs/tacrolimus/#indicationsAndDoses

180 B - Colchicine

NSAIDs can also be used but diclofenac has been advised to be avoided due to adverse cardiovascular events.

https://bnf.nice.org.uk/drugs/colchicine/

181 C - Keratitis

Symptoms are typical of keratitis, patient is a contact lens wearer, she slept in her contact lenses likely causing an abrasion, and she has redness around her iris and has watering discharge.

https://cks.nice.org.uk/topics/red-eye/

182 E - Maxitrol

Maxitrol is a steroid based eye drop usually when prophylactic antibiotic treatment is also required, after excluding the presence of fungal and viral disease.

https://www.medicines.org.uk/emc/product/841/smpc

183 B - Advise the mother that otitis media is self-limiting, and he should continue with paracetamol. Symptoms can take 3–7 days to resolve and if her son's symptoms persists or worsens to see a GP

It is not A because ear calm is for otitis externa and not appropriate for this patient. It is not C because the patient is asthmatic and therefore cannot take ibuprofen. It is not D because it does not need A and E input. It is not E because the patient doesn't require antibiotics at this stage, it is only indicated if patient is systemically unwell.

https://cks.nice.org.uk/topics/otitis-media-acute/

184 C - Glandosane aerosol spray

Glandosane aerosol spray as this is artificial saliva.

https://bnf.nice.org.uk/medical-devices/artificial-saliva-products/glandosane/

185 D - 100g

See BNF for suitable quantities of corticosteroid preparations to be prescribed for specific areas of the body.

https://bnf.nice.org.uk/treatment-summaries/topical-corticosteroids/

186 C- 2 - 8°C.

Care must be taken to store all vaccines under the conditions recommended in the product literature, otherwise the preparation may become ineffective. Refrigerated storage is usually necessary; many vaccines need to be stored at 2–8°C and not allowed to freeze.

https://bnf.nice.org.uk/treatment-summaries/vaccination-general-principles/

187 A – Anaesthetics

As these are the active ingredients.

https://bnf.nice.org.uk/drugs/lidocaine-with-prilocaine/#patient-and-carer-advice

ANSWERS

188 E - Sildenafil

Erectile dysfunction is a very common side effect of goserelin.
https://www.medicines.org.uk/emc/product/1543/smpc

189 B - Book an appointment with the GP, so he can review symptoms and make a 2-week referral to cancer pathway

According to BNF/NICE, there are a few red flags here. This patient is over the age of 55 years with new onset dyspepsia. The GP would have to explore whether this is unexplained or can be linked to changes in the patient's diet/lifestyle. Unexplained dyspepsia in patients over the age of 55 years old is a red flag. Dyspepsia in patients over the age of 55 that is associated with alarming features such as pain, unintentional weight loss or difficulty swallowing is also a red flag and requires urgent investigation via endoscopy. In primary care, urgent referrals are usually seen within 2 weeks to rule out something more sinister such as cancer.
https://cks.nice.org.uk/topics/dyspepsia-unidentified-cause/

190 B - Short course of lowest most effective dose of naproxen

As per the pain ladder, this patient is already using two first line options to treat her pain, e.g. paracetamol and a topical NSAID. The next step is to try a short course of either an NSAID (oral) or COX-2 at the lowest effective dose. It is important to emphasise that these are short course or to be used 'when required' to prevent long term implications of both of these classes of medication. In practice it is common to see that patients have not been counselled on this and end up taking this regularly long term.
https://www.nice.org.uk/Guidance/CG177

191 G - Urgent referral to A&E

A complication of contact lens use is corneal ulceration and microbial keratitis which can be due to poor lens use or care. This is usually presented as unilateral pain and redness and requires urgent referral to remove the contact lens.
https://cks.nice.org.uk/topics/red-eye/diagnosis/diagnosis/

192 F - Treat with over the counter product

Using either the FEVERPAIN or Centor Criteria to decide if antibiotics are needed for tonsillitis, you will find that this patient has not reached

the required score to be referred to the GP for this. Thus, symptoms can be managed with an OTC product, e.g. lozenges, difflam spray etc.
https://ctu1.phc.ox.ac.uk/feverpain/index.php

193 F - Treat with over the counter product
A wide range of products to help treat head lice can be bought over the counter.
https://cks.nice.org.uk/topics/head-lice/

194 B - The vaccines are both live and should either be administered on the same day or 4 weeks apart, but should preferably be administered on different limbs
As per BNF guidance.
https://bnf.nice.org.uk/treatment-summaries/measles-mumps-and-rubella-vaccine/
https://bnf.nice.org.uk/drugs/bacillus-calmette-guerin-vaccine/

195 B - Long term prednisolone due to the risk of a precipitous fall in blood pressure
This is the only likely risk during this procedure.
https://bnf.nice.org.uk/treatment-summaries/surgery-and-long-term-medication/

196 C - Evening
Optimal effect is obtained if latanoprost eye drops is administered in the evening.
https://bnf.nice.org.uk/drug/latanoprost.html?msclkid=c7dafbfdac3111eca1eea31970bb8598#medicinalForms

197 C - Nasonex allergy control (mometasone) nasal spray
Beconase hayfever (beclometasone) – P. Beconase hayfever relief for adults (beclometasone) – GSL. Nasofan allergy (fluticasone) for adults – P. Pirinase hayfever (fluticasone) – P. Pirinase hayfever relief (fluticasone) for adults – GSL. Pollenase hayfever relief (beclometasone) for adults – GSL. Nasacort allergy relief (triamcinolone) nasal spray – GSL.
Additional information:
Betnesol (betamethasone) drops – POM. Flixonase nasule (fluticasone)

nasal drops – POM. Nasonex allergy control (mometasone) nasal spray – POM. Nasobec aqueous (beclometasone) nasal spray – POM.
https://bnf.nice.org.uk/treatment-summary/nose.html

198 B - Betamethasone valerate 0.025%

Beclometasone dipropionate 0.025% is potent, clobetasol 0.05% is very potent, diflucortolone valerate 0,1% is very potent and hydrocortisone butyrate 0.1% is potent.
https://www.nice.org.uk/guidance/ta81/chapter/appendix-d-topical-corticosteroids-for-the-treatment-of-atopic-eczema-grouped-by-potency?m sclkid=563f653dac6111ec913d9e6bcccffe63

199 D - Pneumococcal polysaccharide vaccine

From 50 years: influenza vaccine (annually after September). From 65 years: pneumococcal polysaccharide vaccine. From 70-79 years: herpes-zoster vaccine.
https://www.nhs.uk/conditions/vaccinations/nhs-vaccinations-and-when-to-have-them/

200 C - Pancuronium bromide

This is an aminosteroid neuromuscular blocking drug with a long duration of action. Atracurium besilate is a benzylisoquinolinium neuromuscular blocking drug with an intermediate duration of action. Mivacurium, a benzylisoquinolinium neuromuscular blocking drug, has a short duration of action. Rocuronium bromide exerts an effect within 2 minutes and has the most rapid onset of any of the non-depolarising neuromuscular blocking drugs. It is an aminosteroid neuromuscular blocking drug with an intermediate duration of action. Vecuronium bromide, an aminosteroid neuromuscular blocking drug, has an intermediate duration of action. Hint: duration of action as short-acting (15–30 minutes), intermediate-acting (30–40 minutes), and long-acting (60–120 minutes).
https://bnf.nice.org.uk/treatment-summary/neuromuscular-blockade. html?msclkid=b1c7390daac311ec9508fad881edc750

201 B - Handing out dispensed medicine to the delivery driver

Activities that can take place only in the physical presence of a pharmacist include:

- Professional check (clinical and legal check) of a prescription
- Sale/supply of P medicines
- Sale/supply of POMs (e.g. handing dispensed medicines to patient, patient representative or a delivery person)
- Supply of medicines under a patient group direction (PGD)
- Wholesale of medicines
- Emergency supply of a medicine(s) at the request of a patient or healthcare professional
- Wasting of patient returned CDs
- Receiving CDs from pharmaceutical wholesalers into the building
https://www.rpharMscom/LinkClick.aspx?fileticket=HKrEo4Xvgqo%3d&portalid=0

202 **B - For 2 years from the date of the last entry**
Registers should be kept for two years from the date of the last entry
https://www.rpharMscom/LinkClick.aspx?fileticket=d13ozFluz1k%3d&portalid=0

203 **A - Human Medicines Regulations (2012)**
https://www.legislation.gov.uk/uksi/2012/1916/part/13/made
https://www.gov.uk/guidance/medicines-packaging-labelling-and-patient-information-leaflets

204 **C - Schedule 3**
As per controlled drug legislation.
https://www.gov.uk/government/news/reclassification-of-pregabalin-and-gabapentin-to-schedule-3-drugs-from-1-april-2019

205 **A - Nurse/midwife**
They can prescribe unlicensed medication.
https://psnc.org.uk/dispensing-supply/receiving-a-prescription/who-can-prescribe-what/

206 **B - Age of the patient if under 16 years**
https://bnf.nice.org.uk/guidance/prescription-writing.html

207 **E - The pharmacist must receive payment for the medication supplied**
https://bnf.nice.org.uk/guidance/emergency-supply-of-medicines.html

208 C – 130g

To cover the areas indicated on the body.

https://bnf.nice.org.uk/treatment-summary/topical-corticosteroids.html

209 A - Apply the same high standards when using social media as used in face-to-face interactions

As a part of professionalism.

https://www.pharmacyregulation.org/standards/standards-for-pharmacy-professionals

210 C - Miss JL should have signed up for the pregnancy prevention programme

This is needed for those who will be taking isotretinoin.

https://bnf.nice.org.uk/drugs/isotretinoin/

211 D - Folic acid tablets

They prevent the risk of spina bifida.

https://bnf.nice.org.uk/drugs/folic-acid/#indications-and-dose

212 E - Hydroxocobalamin IV

For deficiency treatment.

https://bnf.nice.org.uk/drugs/hydroxocobalamin/#indications-and-dose

213 B - Colecalciferol capsules

Vitamin D can be purchased safely over the counter.

https://bnf.nice.org.uk/drugs/colecalciferol/

214 F - Levothyroxine tablets

Due to likely hypothyroidism.

https://bnf.nice.org.uk/drugs/levothyroxine-sodium/

215 G - Thiamine tablets

Uusually prescribed in alcoholism to prevent Wernicke-Korsakoff.

https://bnf.nice.org.uk/drugs/thiamine/

216 C - Croup

Croup (laryngotracheobronchitis) is a common childhood disease that is usually caused by a virus. It is characterized by the sudden onset of a seal-like barking cough usually accompanied by stridor. COVID-19 usually presents with a high tempura, a new or continuous cough or a loss of change in smell or taste, so it is unlikely to be the cause. Cystic fibrosis: clinical features include persistent moist cough and gastrointestinal symptoms that are often present from birth. For the common cold the chest is usually clear on examination. Tuberculosis is usually associated with travel abroad and present with weight loss, night sweats and hemoptysis so it is unlikely to be this.

https://cks.nice.org.uk/topics/croup/diagnosis/diagnosis/

217 B - Fluoxetine

When an antidepressant is prescribed, the selective serotonin re-uptake inhibitor (SSRI) fluoxetine is the first-line treatment in children. Paroxetine, venlafaxine and tricyclic antidepressants should not be used for the treatment of depression in children and young people.

https://bnfc.nice.org.uk/treatment-summaries/
depression/?msclkid=211ced62ac7511eca412a95e97cf4777

218 C - Ibuprofen can be used to manage pain or fever

Paracetamol if pain or fever are causing distress (avoid nonsteroidal anti-inflammatory drugs). Hint: all the other statements are correct and can be used to supplement knowledge.

https://cks.nice.org.uk/topics/chickenpox/management/child-or-adult/

219 A - A 20-year-old patient presenting with a red eye

Conjunctivitis is also known as red or pink eye. There is a risk of grey baby syndrome if chloramphenicol is used in pregnancy (fusidic acid eye drops is safe to use). Bacterial keratitis can occur in contact lens wearers and would need urgent referral to ophthalmology. SmPC advises to refer to doctor for patient presenting with severe pain within the eye and glaucoma (this list is not exhaustive).

https://www.medicines.org.uk/emc/product/612/smpc, https://cks.nice.org.uk/red-eye#!scenario

220 A - A patient who has started a new diabetes (type 1) medication

The conditions eligible for this service are:

• asthma and COPD

- diabetes (Type 2) type 1 not stated
- hypertension
- hypercholesterolaemia
- osteoporosis
- gout
- glaucoma
- epilepsy
- Parkinson's disease
- urinary incontinence/retention
- heart failure
- acute coronary syndromes
- atrial fibrillation
- long term risks of venous thromboembolism/embolism
- stroke/transient ischaemic attack
- coronary heart disease

This list is as of the latest service specification at the time of writing.
https://psnc.org.uk/servicescommissioning/advancedservices/
nms/?msclkid=5cdbfbd1ac7c11ec9fc9afbe00bf14a0

221 B - Fexofenadine 120mg (allevia) tablets

Fexofenadine (allevia) 120mg tablets classification changed from POM to GSL on 22nd December 2020. Oral lidocaine containing products legal status changed from GSL to Pharmacy only (P) medicine. Tamsulosin, orlistat & chloramphenicol were reclassified from POM to a P medication.
https://www.rpharMscom/resources/pharmacy-guides/reclassification-guide

222 A - 31st Dec 2024

Wording on packaging definition:
Best before January 2025: Discard 31/12/2024
Use before end January 2025: Discard 31/01/2025
Use by January 2025: Discard 31/12/2024
Discard after January 2025: Discard 31/01/2025
Expires January 2025: Discard 31/01/2025
http://psnc.org.uk/sheffield-lpc/wp-content/uploads/sites/79/2013/06/
Expiry-Dates-Guidance-Oct-2013.pdf

223 B – Colic

Episodes of irritability, fussing, or crying that begin and end for no apparent reason and last at least three hours a day, at least three days a week, for at least one week, in an infant up to 4 months of age with no evidence of faltering growth.

https://cks.nice.org.uk/topics/colic-infantile/

224 D - Croup

A distinctive feature of croup is the barking cough which will make the harsh sound whilst breathing in. This sound is called stridor.

https://cks.nice.org.uk/topics/croup

225 A - Chickenpox

It is common for patients to have viral symptoms a few days before the rash for chickenpox appears. The cycle of the rash is that they start as tiny red spots, then turn into fluid filled blisters which eventually crust over and turn into scabs.

https://cks.nice.org.uk/topics/chickenpox/

226 G - Meningitis

A red flag symptom that should be ruled out for ANY rash is a non-blanching rash when the glass test is used, which is the classical symptom of meningitis. However, it is not always an early sign and symptoms do not appear in order, thus it is important to look out for other signs and symptoms of patients being systemically unwell.

https://cks.nice.org.uk/topics/meningitis-bacterial-meningitis-meningococcal-disease/

227 C - Loratadine tablets

The eye drops will only treat her itchy eyes, and this patient would like something that will allow her to continue her daily activities so it is important to suggest something all inclusive. Chlorphenamine is a sedating antihistamine and thus may interfere with her studies which seems to be one of her worries so not ideal. Sudafed contains a decongestant used for nasal congestion which the patient hasn't mentioned she is suffering with. Thus, loratadine is the most suitable option.

https://www.medicines.org.uk/emc/product/4501/smpc

228 **D - Lactulose and senna**
In patients with opioid-induced constipation, an osmotic laxative (or docusate sodium) to soften the stools) and a stimulant laxative is recommended. Bulk-forming laxatives should be avoided.
https://bnf.nice.org.uk/treatment-summaries/constipation/

229 **B - Dalivit drops**
All other options in the list are not suitable for patients with nut allergy. Sytron contains just iron and no other vitamins so is also not a suitable recommendation.
http://www.dalivit.co.uk/dalivitspc.html

230 **E - Terbinafine cream**
This is likely athlete's foot.
https://cks.nice.org.uk/topics/fungal-skin-infection-foot/

231 **E - Refer to GP surgery to get a prescription for nystatin oral suspension**
Although miconazole oral gel can be bought OTC, there is a severe interaction between miconazole and warfarin whereby it increases the anticoagulant effect of warfarin. Thus, without close monitoring of INR, this should be avoided (MHRA).
https://www.gov.uk/drug-safety-update/miconazole-daktarin-over-the-counter-oral-gel-contraindicated-in-patients-taking-warfarin

232 **D - You are satisfied that there is an immediate need for the emergency supply**
This is a legal requirement to ensure there is a true need for the patient to obtain the medication. Refer to MEP. Edition 44, Section 3.310, Emergency Supply, Page 74.

233 **B - Add quantity in words or figures if missing in one or the other but not both**
Refer to MEP Edition 44, Section 3.6.7, page 110 or BNF.
https://bnf.nice.org.uk/medicines-guidance/controlled-drugs-and-drug-dependence/

234 **D - The pharmacist can hand out the methadone supply on a day prior the date the pharmacy is closed as long as the prescription contains the specific home office wording**

Refer to MEP Edition 44, Section 3.6.7, page 112-113 or BNF.
https://bnf.nice.org.uk/medicines-guidance/controlled-drugs-and-drug-dependence/

235 E - Set up a telephone consultation with the prescriber to discuss rationale behind the prescribing choice

You should wonder why this was prescribed first-line given that her weight most likely will have contributed to this diagnosis and weight gain is a typical side effect of the pioglitazone. As per the standards for pharmacy professionals, it would be your duty as a pharmacist to:

- Speak up when you have concerns (standard 8)
- Use your professional judgement (standard 5), to suggest a more suitable prescribing choice that will aid weight loss and thus her overall diabetes management.
- Communicate effectively (standard 3). In this scenario a telephone consultation is appropriate. It would be an unrealistic expectation to try to have a face-to-face meeting with the prescriber due to demands in the pharmacy.
- Providing person-centred care (standard 1). Having built a rapport with this patient, you are in a position to recommend a more suitable prescribing choice according to her specific needs/lifestyle.

236 B - In the axilla

This is the most appropriate method of taking the temperature.
https://www.nhs.uk/conditions/baby/health/how-to-take-your-babystemperature/

237 A - Chickenpox

Based on the presentation, the most likely diagnosis is chickenpox because of the spreading fluid filled red lumps on the stomach, itchiness and that otherwise the patient otherwise is well. Often children may have experienced viral symptoms prior to skin presentation.
https://cks.nice.org.uk/topics/chickenpox/

238 C - Glandular fever

Transmitted from close salivary contact, is also known as the 'kissing disease' and has an incubation period of 4 to 7 weeks. Symptoms are

vague but characterised by fatigue, headache, sore throat and swollen and tender lymph glands. A macular rash can also occur in a small proportion of patients. The symptoms tend to be mild but can linger for many months.
https://www.nhs.uk/conditions/glandular-fever/

239 A - Clotrimazole 1% cream
The symptoms suggest that the patient has nappy rash that is candidal in nature. This is since there are lesions, other sites are involved (hands), and it is bright red and well demarcated.
https://cks.nice.org.uk/topics/nappy-rash/

240 A - Dose is incorrect, it should be 50mg three times a day for a 3-month year old

241 C - Fever for 3 days

242 C - Subconjunctival haemorrhage
This is likely a ruptured blood vessel as 'bright red' is used to describe the eye. Patient has a cough and though this can come on spontaneously it also can be precipitated by cough. It is in one eye and not painful, therefore indicative of subconjunctival haemorrhage.
https://cks.nice.org.uk/topics/red-eye/diagnosis/diagnosis/

243 C – Refer to GP
Since the patient is diabetic, considerations need to be made with regards to diabetic foot, e.g. they may require a foot check.
https://cks.nice.org.uk/topics/diabetes-type-2/management/management-adults/

244 D - Permethrin is the first line of choice and a whole tube should be used on everyone in the household as a single application. Some adults may need more than one tube to cover their body.
This is false since a quarter of a tube should be used for those 2 months to 5 years of age. Since the child is 2-years-old, it is important to note that the amount to be used on each patient varies with age. Ensure to consult product literature.
https://www.medicines.org.uk/emc/product/6540/smpc

245 B - Carbamazepine

Phenytoin and carbamazepine decrease mebendazole plasma levels.

https://www.medicines.org.uk/emc/product/975/smpc#INTERACTIONS

246 B - Miss HM, a 25-year-old woman, who works as an air hostess has recently come off night flights and has been put on day flights, which she is struggling with as she can't sleep at night. She is requesting Nytol for a short term to help with her altered sleep pattern.

This is because the patient has an altered sleeping pattern and it is also short term. Scenario A: Nytol cannot be sold in children under 12 so it is best to refer the patient, it could possibly be anxiety. Scenario C: The patient is on fluoxetine which can cause insomnia. They also describe being in pain which may need to be discussed with his GP, so they should be referred to their GP. Scenario D: This has been going on for more than 4 weeks and the patient seems like he may have anxiety or depression therefore needs to be referred. Scenario E: She advises she has been unable to sleep for years which is greater than 4 weeks. It is best to refer them to their GP.

247 E - Ketoconazole 2% cream

Ketoconazole 2% cream is not licensed in patients with vulvovaginal candidiasis.

https://www.medicines.org.uk/emc/product/970/smpc

248 B - Co-amoxiclav

Broad spectrum antibiotics can contribute to yeast infections in patients by altering normal flora.

https://bnf.nice.org.uk/drugs/co-amoxiclav/

249 C - Rabeprazole

Rabeprazole is a POM medication, the rest can be purchased over the counter.

https://bnf.nice.org.uk/drugs/rabeprazole-sodium/

250 C - Plaque psoriasis

Plaque psoriasis is commonly associated with scaling and thickening therefore most likely diagnosis.

https://cks.nice.org.uk/topics/psoriasis/

ANSWERS

251 D - Paracetamol PO 1g QDS

The patient has asthma and hypertension as per her medication, NSAIDs are therefore not appropriate. A trial of paracetamol is the best treatment plan and referral onward failing that.

252 D - Loratadine

The patient is a bus driver and so requires a non-drowsy preparation. The most appropriate would be loratadine as it is non-drowsy.
https://www.medicines.org.uk/emc/product/4501/smpc

253 E - Tension

This is since it is described as frontal and tightness, like a weight is pressing down on it which is all indicative of tension type headaches. Frontal: tension or migraine. Orbital: cluster, glaucoma and sinusitis. Occipital: subarachnoid haemorrhage, tension. Temporal: migraine, temporal arteritis.
https://cks.nice.org.uk/topics/headache-tension-type/

254 C - Guafanesin

Used for patients with a productive cough. The patient does not attend with anything that requires GP referral at this stage. Glycerin, honey and lemon, pholcodine and dextromethorphan are commonly used for a dry cough.
https://cks.nice.org.uk/topics/cough/management/management/

255 C - Refer patient to GP as codeine containing products are restricted to a short-term (3 days) treatment of acute pain

Codeine containing products are restricted to a short-term (3 days) treatment of acute, moderate pain, which is not relieved by paracetamol, ibuprofen, or aspirin alone. (See MHRA guidance).
https://www.chemistanddruggist.co.uk/CD011648/MHRA-introduces-new-codeine-restrictions

256 D - The number of gabapentin capsules to be dispensed is not allowed

The number of gabapentin capsules to be dispensed is not allowed. This is since gabapentin is a controlled drug and the number given should not exceed 30 days. (Controlled drug legislation – see MEP Edition 44, Section 3.6.7, page 111)

257 **A - 28 days** (See MEP Edition 44, Section 3.6.7, page 110)

258 **E - Written or printed legibly in indelible ink**
The weight of the patient where it has been used to determine dose. The rest are considered legal requirements for prescription writing.
https://bnf.nice.org.uk/medicines-guidance/prescription-writing/

259 **B - Schedule 2**
Any person who purchases or supplies any product containing a CD specified in Schedule 2 must maintain a Controlled Drugs Register (CDR).

260 **A - Displaying a notice that gives the details of who the responsible pharmacist is**
This is a legal requirement as per The Medicines Act.
https://www.pharmacyregulation.org/responsible-pharmacist

261 **D- Reflect on feedback or concerns, taking action as appropriate and thinking about what can be done to prevent the same thing from happening again**
See GPhC professional standards.
https://www.pharmacyregulation.org/standards/standards-for-pharmacy-professionals

262 **B - Refer to GP**
Refer to GP, the patient needs antihistamines but none are licensed for sale and supply due to age (most likely chickenpox). Piriton is not licensed under the age of 1, loratadine is 2 years.
https://cks.nice.org.uk/topics/chickenpox/

263 **D - Take a further dose after 2 weeks if reinfection is suspected**
This is recommended as good practice - see PIL and SPC.
https://www.medicines.org.uk/emc/product/975#gref

264 **B - If ellaOne is supplied, then you must inform the patient to continue with barrier methods until the next period**
Barrier methods until the next menses is relevant to ellaOne only.
https://www.medicines.org.uk/emc/product/6657/smpc#gref

265 **D - Omeprazole may be trialled first-line**

Option appropriate for the baby.

https://bnfc.nice.org.uk/treatment-summary/gastro-oesophageal-reflux-disease.html

266 **E - The most appropriate add-on therapy is inhaled beclomethasone 100mg twice daily**

The patient is using her SABA quite frequently.

https://cks.nice.org.uk/topics/asthma/

267 **E - You should advise Mr LD to resign from his job to optimise his health**

He does not need to leave his job, he can take measures to help manage his symptoms.

https://cks.nice.org.uk/topics/irritable-bowel-syndrome/
https://bnf.nice.org.uk/drug/peppermint-oil.html

268 **F – Tinnitus**

Due to symptoms such as humming.

https://cks.nice.org.uk/topics/tinnitus/

269 **A - Ear wax**

Due to symptoms such as fullness.

https://cks.nice.org.uk/topics/earwax/

270 **C - Otitis media**

Due to symptoms and examination findings.

https://cks.nice.org.uk/topics/otitis-media-acute/

271 **E – Sinusitis**

Due to symptoms e.g. frontal headache.

https://cks.nice.org.uk/topics/sinusitis/

272 **B - Otitis externa**

Due to symptoms e.g. itch and history includes she is a swimmer.

https://cks.nice.org.uk/topics/otitis-externa/diagnosis/

273 F - Movicol paediatric sachets

No bowel movement for 10 days so needs something that will work effectively, query impaction.

https://bnf.nice.org.uk/drugs/macrogol-3350/

274 E - Lactulose liquid

Can be sold over the counter safely to this patient.

https://bnf.nice.org.uk/drugs/lactulose/

275 A - Bisacodyl suppository

The patient is requesting quick acting formulation.

https://bnf.nice.org.uk/drugs/bisacodyl/#indications-and-dose

276 C - Fleet ready to use enema

This is used for bowel evacuation prior to a procedure.

https://bnf.nice.org.uk/drugs/sodium-acid-phosphate-with-sodium-phosphate/#indications-and-dose

277 D - Fybogel sachets

Important counselling regarding Fybogel when supplying or prescribing to a patient who will take this for the first time.

https://bnf.nice.org.uk/drugs/ispaghula-husk/

278 H - Simple analgesia

https://cks.nice.org.uk/topics/hand-foot-mouth-disease/

279 C - Dexamethasone PO stat

https://cks.nice.org.uk/topics/croup/

280 A - Admit to hospital

Potentially life threatening so needs to be admitted.

https://cks.nice.org.uk/topics/meningitis-bacterial-meningitis-meningococcal-disease/

281 H - Simple analgesia

https://cks.nice.org.uk/topics/otitis-media-acute/

282 G - Prescribe antifungals as per local guidance

https://cks.nice.org.uk/topics/threadworm/

283 E - Adrenaline IM auto-injector 0.3mg

https://bnfc.nice.org.uk/drug/adrenalineepinephrine.html

284 A - Prednisolone soluble 5mg tablets, 6 tablets daily for 7 days

https://bnf.nice.org.uk/drug/prednisolone.html

285 A - 200mg bd

286 A - Do not supply ibuprofen

Avoid in chickenpox due to risk of skin infection.

https://www.nhs.uk/conditions/chickenpox/

287 B – Dizziness

The only antimuscuranic listed side effect.

https://bnf.nice.org.uk/drugs/amitriptyline-hydrochloride/

288 D – Pantoprazole

Proton pump inhibitors can mask the symptoms of gastric cancer.

https://bnf.nice.org.uk/drugs/pantoprazole/

289 E - Trial low dose omeprazole

Can safely prescribe in this pregnant patient.

https://bnf.nice.org.uk/drugs/omeprazole/#indications-and-dose

290 C - Lansoprazole

Lansoprazole can cause low magnesium levels

https://www.medicines.org.uk/emc/product/4164

291 A - Copper intrauterine device

A copper device would be the most appropriate in this case as the patient has poor compliance so A would not be a good choice. C and E are HRT therapy and D is a combined pill which is not appropriate due to her risk factors.

https://bnf.nice.org.uk/treatment-summaries/contraceptives-hormonal/

292 E - 6.25ml daily
100mcg/5ml therefore 25mcg/1.25ml = 6.25ml

293 D - All of the above
They are all drugs that induce hepatic enzyme activity.
https://bnf.nice.org.uk/treatment-summaries/contraceptives-interactions/

294 C - Prescribe NSAID and antibiotics
As this could be mastitis.
https://cks.nice.org.uk/topics/mastitis-breast-abscess/management/

295 A - Can restart sertraline
SSRIs are usually safest to take during lactation. Mrs BW was doing well on sertraline prior to giving birth so would be appropriate to restart.
https://www.sps.nhs.uk/articles/safety-in-lactation-antidepressants/

296 B - Gliclazide
The sulfonylureas (glibenclamide, gliclazide, glimepiride, glipizide, tolbutamide) may cause hypoglycaemia; it is more likely with long-acting sulfonylureas such as glibenclamide, which have been associated with severe, prolonged and sometimes fatal cases of hypoglycaemia.
https://bnf.nice.org.uk/drugs/gliclazide/#indications-and-dose

297 C - 65mg
Ferrous sulfate 200 mg is equivalent to 65 mg iron.
https://bnf.nice.org.uk/drugs/ferrous-sulfate/

298 A - Hyperkalaemia
Monitor electrolytes and discontinue if hyperkalaemia occurs.
https://bnf.nice.org.uk/drugs/spironolactone/

299 C - 8
Since 4 drops equate to 10mg tablet, 8 drops equate to 20mg.

300 A - Schedule 1
Pharmacist are allowed to be in possession of CD in schedule 2 – 5 when acting in their capacity as a pharmacist.
MEP Edition 44, Section 3.63, pg 106.

Calculations answers

301 21 vials

Note: do ensure you are using correct units - BSA is calculated using height in centimetres. Using the formula given, BSA = 1.66 m^2

Dose = 1.66m^2 × 15mg = 24.8mg = 3 vials/day (available as 10mg vials)

3 vials × 7 days = 21 vials

302 0.056L

C1 × V1 = C2 × V2

1 in 4000 = 0.025% w/v (C2) (Please note 1% w/v = 1g/100ml (percentage weight in volume))

0.025 × 50 (dilution factor) = 1.25 (C1)

200ml × 2 × 7 days = 2,800 ml (V2)

C1 × V1 = C2 × V2

1.25 × ? = 0.025 × 2,800

70 ÷ 1.25 = 56ml

? = 56ml = 0.056L

303 8.4g

25 × 20/100 = 5 (surplus)

Total suppository is 30

30 × 300mg = 9000mg = 9g

30 × 40mg = 1200mg = 1.2g

DV of 2 means 2g of drug displaces 1g of theobroma oil base

Therefore 1.2 grams of drug must displace 0.6 grams of base

9g – 0.6g = 8.4g

304 **£230**

30 × 90/100 = 27 patients eligible

Drug X: £34.55 ÷ 28 tabs × 30 days = £37.02 (round at pence) × 3 × 27
          = £2,998.62

Drug Z: £31.95 ÷ 28 tabs × 30 days = £34.23 (round at pence) × 3 × 27
          = £2,772.63

£2,998.62 – £2,772.63 = £225.99 = £230 (nearest £10)

OR

Saving per patient per 30-day period: £37.02 – £34.23 = £2.79

Saving over 3 repeats per patient: £2.79 × 3 = £8.37

Saving for total number patients: £8.37 × 27 = £225.99 = £230 (nearest £10)

305 **30 tablets**

8 days of treatment left (not quantity of medication left!).

Longest duration of medication will last 28 days, therefore 20 days' worth of furosemide is needed to synchronise the medication.

20 days = 30 tablets (at a dose of take 3 tabs daily)

306 **226 mins**

0.8ml × 40kg = 32ml ÷ 60 × 30 = 16ml ⎫
1.2ml × 40kg = 48ml ÷ 60 × 40 = 32ml ⎬ Total: 108ml
1.8ml × 40kg = 72ml ÷ 60 × 50 = 60ml ⎭

0.8g × 40 = 32g

10% (10g/100ml) = 32g/320ml (total volume infused)

320ml – 108ml = 212ml

3ml × 40kg ÷ 60mins = 2ml/min

212ml ÷ 2ml = 106min

106 + 30 + 40 + 50 minutes = 226 minutes

307 **0.55ml**

Day 1 (prior) = 3 drops

Day 2 (surgery day) = 4 drops (with additional drop)

Postoperative (14 days × 3 drops) = 42 drops

Total drops used = 49 drops

49 drops / 20 drops = 2.45ml used

3ml – 2.45ml = 0.55ml

308 58.5%

1mmol= 58.5mg (Moles = Mass/Mr)

3mmol = 175.5mg (1 sachet)

20 (sachet) = 3,510mg = 3.51g

3,510mg/6000mg (daily intake) (or 3.51g/6g) × 100 = 58.5%

309 45.5ml/min

BMI = weight (kg) / height (m2)

88kg/2.81 = 31.3kg/m2

BMI >30 therefore must use IBW

IBW = 50 + (2.3 × 6) = 63.8kg

Using the Cockcroft and Gault formula

CrCl = 45.49 = 45.5ml/min (rounded to one decimal place)

310 2400 minutes

4480mg/L = 0 hours

2240mg/L = 4 hours

1120mg/L = 8 hours

560mg/L = 12 hours

280mg/L = 16 hours

140mg/L = 20 hours

70mg/L = 24 hours

35mg/L = 28 hours

17.5mg/L = 32 hours

8.75mg/L = 36 hours

4.375mg/L (4,375 mcg/L) = 40 hours

40 hours × 60 mins = 2400 minutes

311 210 tablets

Strength (Reduce by 2.5mg every 2 weeks)	Number of tablets	Number of tablets in 2 weeks	Number of 2.5mg tablets needed
15mg	15/2.5 = 6	6 × 14 = 84	Given by Dermatology
12.5mg	12.5/2.5 = 5	5 × 14 = 70	70
10mg	10/2.5 = 4	4 × 14 = 56	56
7.5mg	7.5/2.5=3	3 × 14 = 42	42
5mg	5/2.5=2	2 × 14 = 28	28
2.5mg	2.5/2.5=1	1 × 14 = 14	14
STOP	STOP	STOP	0
TOTAL			210 tablets needed

312 **4.5ml**

Dose: 30mg/kg three times a day

Weight: 7.5kg

Therefore: $30mg \times 7.5$ – three times a day

$\qquad$ = 225mg – three times day

Strength of suspension: 250mg in 5ml

The question asks how many ml in each dose

So if there is 250mg in 5ml

Then there is 5/250mg in 1ml

So in 225mg the equation would be

$5/250 \times 225mg = 4.5ml$ in each dose

313 **Oxycontin 20mg twice a day**

Patient currently receiving: morphine m/r 30mg twice a day = m/r 60mg daily

10mg m/r morphine = 6.6mg m/r oxycodone

1mg $\qquad$ = 6.6mg / 10

60mg $\qquad$ = 6.6mg/ 10×60

$\qquad$ = 39.6mg oxycodone which is equivalent to 40mg daily

Since modified release doses are given as twice a day – 40mg / 2 = 20mg

314 **195 tablets for the whole course**

Onset: 21st April

3 days before onset (18th, 19th and 20th April) – $3 \times 3 \times 5 = 45$

Menstruation occurs: 2 – 3 days after stopping

If we say 2 days after – as the question asks maximum number of 5mg tablets

Question states patient doesn't mind coming on any time on or after 2nd

so tablets need to be given up until 30th April.

(21st, 22nd, 23rd, 24th, 25th, 26th, 27th, 28th, 29th, 30th - 10days)

$10 \times 3 \times 5 = 150$

3 days before onset + during holiday up until 2 days before pt happy to

have her onset = whole course

$45 + 150 = 195$

315 10ml

BNF states: For Priadel liquid: lithium citrate tetrahydrate 520 mg is equivalent to lithium carbonate 204 mg.

Use ratios:

Priadel tablet (mg): Priadel Liquid (mg)

204mg:520mg

(Divide 204 by itself to simplify the ratio)

1:2.54

So for 400mg tablet: 400mg × 2.54 oral solution

$$= 1016mg$$

So if there 520mg in 5ml

Then there is 5/520mg in 1ml

5/520mg*1016mg = 9.76ml equivalent to 10ml (to the nearest ml as per question)

316 6 drops per day

2740iu in 1ml

1iu in 1 ml / 2750

400iu in 1 / 2750 × 400

= 0.15ml

41 drops in 1ml

41/1 × 0.15 in 0.15ml

= 5.98 – equivalent to 6 drops

317 630ml

Oral Solution: carbocisteine 250mg in 5ml

carbocisteine 1mg in 5ml / 250

carbocisteine 375mg in 5ml/250 × 375

= 7.5ml

Dose: 375mg (7.5ml) three times a day

Daily Dose: 7.5ml × 3 = 22.5ml

Monthly Dose: 22.5 × 28 = 630ml

318 **2.2ml daily**

0.7 = 70% - 70% of tablet dose is available

So 70% of tablet dose is effective which is $70/100 \times 125 = 87.5$

Patient in effect is taking 87.5mcg of the available digoxin dose daily

0.8 = 80% - 80% of oral solution dose is available

The oral solution has a bioavailability of 0.8

If 87.5mcg is the whole availability then the amount or oral solution needed is:

87.5 / 0.8 = 109.3 which is equivalent to 110mcg

If the oral solution is available at 50mcg/ml

50mcg in 1ml

1mcg in 1/50ml

110mcg in $1/50 \times 110 = 2.2$ml

319 **42 drops/min**

Drip rate =

Volume needed (in ml) × drop factor (no. of drops per ml given over the set) / duration of the infusion (minutes)

Note the drip rate is required in drops/min

Therefore

4 hours = 4×60 (min) = 240mins

Drip rate = 500×20 / 240 = 41.67 to nearest decimal – 42 drops/min

320 **7.2ml will be infused in each dose**

BNF - By intravenous infusion for adult (body weight up to 50 kg)

15 mg/kg every 4–6 hours, dose to be administered over 15 minutes

Max dose per day - 15mg/kg every 4 hours

Patient weight = 48kg

Max dose – $15 \times 48 = 720$mg per dose

Amps available as 1g in 10ml = 1000mg in 10ml

1000mg in 10ml

1mg in 10/1000

720mg in $10/1000 \times 720$

321 **15.7**

Simply put in the figures into the equation

CrCl = 140 – age × weight × 1.23 / serum creatinine

CrCl = 140 – 79 × 65 × 1.23 / 264

= 18.47

Since she is a woman

18.47 × 0.85

CrCl = 15.7 to one decimal place

322 **81**

You need to work out the patients age

CrCl = 140 – age × weight × 1.23 / serum creatinine

29.9 = (140 – age) × 81 × 1.23 / 196

29.9 = (140 – age) × 99.63 / 196

29.9 = 13978.2 × 99.63age / 196

29.9 = 71.16 – 0.508age

29.9 – 71.16 = - 0.508age

29.9 – 71.16 / - 0.508 = age

81 = age

Age = 81 to nearest number

323 **77kg**

You need to work out the patient's weight

CrCl = 140 – age × weight × 1.23 / serum creatinine

85.4 = 140 – 67 × weight × 1.23/81

85.4 = 89.79weight/81

85.4 × 81 = 89.79weight

6917.4 = 89.79weight

6917.4 / 89.79 = weight

77 = weight

Weight = 77kg to nearest number

324 **Female**

Is it a male or female, this is deduced through putting the numbers in the equation in, if the numbers when plugged in matches the creatinine clearance then it is male, if however the numbers only match when multiplied by 0.85 then it is a female.

CrCl = 140 – age × weight × 1.23 / serum creatinine
   = 140 – 61 × 54 × 1.23 / 288
   = 18.2

This does not match the figure given

18.2 × 0.85 = 15.4

This does match the figure given therefore the patient is female

325 Need to work out patients serum creatinine (mmol/l)

CrCl = 140 – age × weight × 1.23 / serum creatinine

109.9 = 140 – 54 × 79 × 1.23/ serum creatinine

109.9 = 8356.62 / serum creatinine

109.9 × serum creatinine = 8356.62

serum creatinine = 8356.62 / 109.9

serum creatinine = 76

326 420 tablets

Weaning to start in 4 weeks

5× 1mg= 5 tablets/day

5 tablets × 7 days = 35 tablets/week

35 tablets × 4 weeks = 140 tablets (on 5mg)

4× 1mg =4 tablets /day

4 tablets × 7 days= 28 tablets/week

28 tablets × 4 weeks= 112 tablets (on 4mg)

3×1mg= 3 tablets/day

3 tablets × 7 days= 21 tablets / week

21 tablets × 4 weeks= 84 tablets (on 3mg)

2 tablets × 1mg- 2 tablets/day

2 tablets × 7 days= 14 tablets/week

14 tablets × 4 weeks = 56 tablets (on 2mg)

1 × 1mg = 1 tablet/day

1 tablet × 7 days = 7 tablets/week

7 tablets × 4 weeks= 28 tablets (on 1mg)

140+112+84+56+28= 420

327 3 pens

10 units +12 units = 22 units/ day

22 units × 28 days= 616 units needed for 1 month supply

100 units/ ml and each pen contain 3ml= 300 units

616 units= 6.16 ml/ month = 3 pens

328 **4 packs**

1.25g contains 0.75mg estradiol

Therefore, 5g contains 3mg estradiol

One 80g pack /5g = 16 days

56 days would require 3.5 packs and thus a total of 4 packs needed (cannot split pack)

329 **15 miligrams**

0.05grams of clobetasone in 100 grams

50 milligrams of clobetasone in 100 grams (divide by 1000 to convert gram to milligram)

15 Milligrams of clobetasone in 30 grams (ensure each side are in the same units and divide 100grams by 3.3 to get 30 grams and do the same to the quantity of clobetasone)

330 **56mg**

112 × 5mg and 56 × 1mg

Dose reduction =

25mg in 4 days = 20 5mg tabs

24mg next 4 days = 16 5mg tabs, 16 1mg tabs

23mg next 4 day = 16 5mg tabs, 12 1mg tabs

22mg next 4 days = 16 5mg tabs, 8 1mg tabs

21mg next 4 days = 16 5mg tabs, 4 1mg tabs

20mg next 4 days = 16 5mg tabs

19mg next 4 days = 12 5mg tabs, 16 1mg tabs

28 days reached

5mg strength = 20+16+16+16+16+16+12 = 112

1mg strength – 16+12+8+4+16 = 56

331 **0.056ml/hour**

BNF = for child 1 month–11 years

0.5–1 mg/kg every 8 hours (max. per dose 40 mg) as required,

1*4.5 = 4.5mg/ 8 hours

20mg/2ml injections available

4.5mg needed therefore 0.45ml

0.45ml divided by 8 = 0.056ml/hour

332 3 packs

Dose = 250mcg QDS = 4 per day = 28 doses for 1 week and 56 doses for 2 weeks

20 nebules in 1 pack therefore 3 packs (60 doses) to cover 2 weeks

333 3 bottles

Usually 20 drops in 1 ml

1 drop 6 times per day in 1 eye = 42 drops per week = 252 drops in six weeks

Therefore 3 bottles needed

334 224 tablets

25mg for 2 weeks = 5*7*2 = 70

20mg for 2 weeks = 4*7*2 = 56

15mg for 2 weeks = 3 *7*2 = 42

10mg for 2 weeks = 2*7*2 = 28

5mg for 4 weeks = 1 *7*4 = 28

335 14,2320

Work out packs per year = 13 (364 days)

Pregablin 150mg 2 BD = 112 capsules per month = 128.80 per month = 2189.6 per pt per month

Pregabalin 300mg 1 BD = 56 capsules per month = 64.40 per month = 1094.8 per pt per month

1545.60 * 13 = 28,464.8

772.8*13 = 14,232.4

28,464.8 – 14,232.4 = 14,232.4 = 14,2320

336 28 tablets

$4 \times 7 = 28$

337 168 sachets

2 sachets per feed as per weight = 2*3 (as has 3 bottled per day) = 6 per day therefore 6 *7*4 = 168 sachets

338 **183ml**

3 weeks

58mg bd for the 1st week, 116mg mane and 58mg pm for the 2nd week, 116mg bd for the 3rd week

812mg week 1, 1218mg week 2, 1624mg week 3

3 weeks = 3654mg = 182.7ml = 183ml

339 **4 tins**

(2 scoops = 2.8g per dose * 5 = 14g per day). 392 grams total for 28 days. Works out to 3.1 tins but will need to supply 4 tins to cover the script.

340 **250mg strength for each dose**

SmPC states: switching from oral formulations to suppositories the dosage should be increased by approximately 25%

Usual dose is 800mg, therefore increasing by 25% gives a new daily dose of 1000mg to be administered via suppository.

1000/4 (dose to be given four times a day) = 250mg strength suppository per individual dose.

341 **80.8ml**

The displacement volume = the volume occupied by a solute when added to a solution.

The final concentration needed is 3mg/ml, therefore 83.3ml is needed for 250mg of drug.

If 50mg displaces 0.5ml of solution, this means 250mg would displace 2.5ml.

83.3ml –2.5ml = 80.8ml

342 **47.26g**

2.6g bismuth displacement value means it can displaces 1g base

24*2g =48g (total suppository number)

0.08 * 24 = 1.92g (total bismuth for all suppositories)

1 / 2.6 *1.92 (to factor in displacement) = 0.73846154

48g-0.73846154 = 47.26g

343 9.5% w/v

Dilution between intermediate and footwash is 20 therefore 20 * 0.475% = 9.5%

344 20ml

Iron need = 1500mg
Single dose should not exceed 20mg/kg therefore 2 doses needed
20ml for 1000mg dose

345 12mg/mL

Final solution is 0.06% = 0.06g in 100ml.
60mg in 100ml
60 divided by 5 = 12mg/ml
OR
The dilution factor, e.g. 100ml divided by 5ml = dilution factor of 20
0.06% × 20 = 1.2% w/v (stock solution in %w/v)
1.2% w/v means 1.2g/100ml
1.2g/100ml = 12mg/1ml

346 0.0015ml/min

BNF – continuous dose = 60mcg/kg/hour = 60mcg × 3kg = 180mcg
180mcg ÷ 60 mins = 3mcg per mins
available as 100mg/50ml = 100,000mcg/50ml
3 microgram ÷ 100,000mcg × 50ml = 0.0015ml/min

347 44.4ml

Dose = 17.4 * 300 divided by 3 = 1740mg = 17.4g
Vial is 2g/30 therefore only one needed
Section 6.6 = Displacement value of fosfomycin 2g is 1ml
2g vial is reconstituted with 20ml and then further 30ml solvent (50ml)
So for DV = 2000mg in 51ml = 39.2157 mg/ml
Volume per dose = 1740mg divided by 39.2157mg/ml = 44.4ml

348 **33000mg**

The BNF extract states zinc and coal tar paste, BP consists of zinc oxide 6%, coal tar 6%, emulsifying wax 5%, starch 38%, yellow soft paraffin 45%.

500g plus 10% excess = 550g

Zinc oxide = 6%

6% of 550 = 33g

33g to mg = 33000mg

349 **2,201mg**

K + Cl = 39.1+35.5 = 74.6

39.1/74.6*4200mg = 2,201.3mg

= 2,201mg

350 **4.4ml**

Total daily dose = 13.2 * 25mg * 4 = 1320mg

Need 4.4ml daily

351 **120ml**

2mmol / 5ml = 4mmol / 10ml = 12mmol / 30ml = 120mmol / 300ml – 0.12moles

Mass = Moles * Mr = 0.12*84 = 10.08

8.4% = 8.4 in 100

100 * 10.08 / 8.4 = 120ml

352 **1.61ml**

Initially 70mcg/kg once daily = 1610 micrograms = 1.61mg OD

5mg/5ml = 1.61mg in 1.61ml

353 **33mg/ml**

2g in 60ml = 3.3g / 100ml = 3300mg/100ml = 33mg/ml

354 **0.4ml/minute**

BNF states max 4mg / minute for doses over 80mg.

20mg/2ml

2mg/0.2ml

Therefore 0.4ml / minute

355 **4 vials**

The SPC shows:

Serum digoxin concentration known

Full neutralisation dose of DIGIFAB is: Number of vials = [serum digoxin concentration (ng/mL) × weight (kg)] / 100 Round up to the nearest vial To calculate the number of milligrams to be prescribed: multiply the number of vials by 40 (as there are 40 mg/vial).

6.3 *63.9 / 100 = 4 vials

356 **200ml**

400ml diluted 1 in 50 = 20,000ml final solution

1 in 250 = 1g in 250ml = 4g in 1,000ml

20,000ml will contain 80g

80g in the original 400ml

The stock solution is 40 % w/v = 40g in 100ml = 4g in 10ml = 80g in 200ml stock needed

OR

c1 × ? = C2 × v2

1 in 250 = 0.4 %w/v

C2 = 0.4 × 50 (dilution factor) = 20

20 × 400 ÷ 40 (available concentrate) = 200ml (C1)

357 **580ml**

0.06 % = 0.06g in 100ml = 0.006g in 10ml = 0.012g in 20ml

20ppm = 20g in 1,000,000ml = 5g in 250,000ml = 1g in 50,000ml = 0.01g in 500ml = 0.001g in 50ml = 0.012g in 600ml

OR

c1 × v1 = c2 × v2

20ppm = 20g/1000,000 = 0.002% w/v (C2)

0.06 × 20ml ÷ 0.002 = 600ml (v2)

600ml - 20ml = 580ml (needed to dilute the concentration)

358 **50 capsules**

BSA = 1.97

Dose = 1.97*240 = daily = 474mg per day

Capsules available as 50mg strength = 10 caps per day (rounded up)

5 day course = 50 capsules

359 21.9g

10 % excess = 11 suppositories

Theoretical mass of base = 11 × 2 = 22g of theobroma oil

Amount of base displaced = (11 × 0.015)/1.5 = 0.11g

Mass of base= 22 - 0.11= 21.89g = 21.9g

360 11 ampoules

2.5mg * 6 = 15mg in 24 hours

15mg * 7 = 105mg in 1 week

10mg in 1 ampoule therefore 11 needed for 1 week

11 ampoules

Further answers

361 A - Cluster headache
Due to symptoms presented by patient (unilateral, duration and pattern).
https://cks.nice.org.uk/topics/headache-cluster/diagnosis/clinical-features/

362 C - Migraine with aura
Due to symptoms presented e.g. visual disturbances with aura.
https://cks.nice.org.uk/topics/migraine/

363 G - Subarachnoid haemorrhage
Due to the thunderclap nature.
https://cks.nice.org.uk/topics/headache-assessment/diagnosis/headache-diagnosis/

364 H - Tension headache
Due to symptoms such as pressing feeling.
https://cks.nice.org.uk/topics/headache-tension-type/

365 E - Side effect of medication
This can occur with amlodipine.
https://bnf.nice.org.uk/drugs/amlodipine/

366 B – Carbamazepine
This is the optimum plasma drug concentration.
https://bnf.nice.org.uk/drugs/carbamazepine/

367 B – Carbamazepine
Due to the risk of blood, hepatic or skin disorders.
https://bnf.nice.org.uk/drugs/carbamazepine/

ANSWERS

368 **A – Amiodarone**

Due to the risk of corneal microdeposits.

https://bnf.nice.org.uk/drugs/amiodarone-hydrochloride/#patient-and-carer-advice

369 **A – Amiodarone**

Sunscreen recommended during treatment.

https://bnf.nice.org.uk/drugs/amiodarone-hydrochloride/#patient-and-carer-advice

370 **D – Lithium**

Changes in sodium levels can alter lithium levels.

https://bnf.nice.org.uk/drugs/lithium-carbonate/#patient-and-carer-advice

371 **C - The CPCS can expect referrals from NHS 111**

This is part of the agreed service.

https://psnc.org.uk/services-commissioning/advanced-services/community-pharmacist-consultation-service/

372 **B - Platelet counts should ideally be checked prior to treatment dose**

Due to risk of heparin-induced thrombocytopenia.

https://bnf.nice.org.uk/drugs/dalteparin-sodium/

373 **B - Irregular pupil size**

This is a red flag.

374 **B - The NMS service covers patients with osteoporosis**

https://psnc.org.uk/services-commissioning/advanced-services/nms/

375 **C – Clopidogrel**

Usually prescribed long term post event.

https://www.nice.org.uk/guidance/ng128

376 **F – Rivaroxaban**

Once daily dosing and no INR monitoring.

https://www.medicines.org.uk/emc/medicine/25586#gref

377 A – Apixaban

Due to routine monitoring: weight, creatinine, age (dose dependent).
https://www.medicines.org.uk/emc/product/13686/smpc

378 E – Fondaparinux

It is suitable for vegetarians.

379 H – Warfarin

Skin reactions can occur.
https://bnf.nice.org.uk/drugs/warfarin-sodium/#indications-and-dose

380 C - Counsel patient on the risks of hypoglycaemia and hyperglycaemia

https://bnf.nice.org.uk/treatment-summaries/beta-adrenoceptor-blocking-drugs/

381 B - Pravastatin

Statin medication can cause muscular aches and pains. Patients are at a higher risk of muscle toxicity such as myopathy or rhabdomyolysis.
https://bnf.nice.org.uk/drugs/pravastatin-sodium/

382 A - The cholesterol level is high thus the patient requires a statin after a lifestyle intervention/discussion

Need to discuss with patient.
https://cks.nice.org.uk/topics/cvd-risk-assessment-management/management/cvd-risk-assessment/

383 F – Perindopril

Do not prescribe if patient has had a history of angioedema to ace inhibitors.
https://bnf.nice.org.uk/drugs/perindopril-arginine/

384 A – Atenolol

Water-soluble beta-blockers (such as atenolol, celiprolol hydrochloride, nadolol, and sotalol hydrochloride) are less likely to enter the brain, and may therefore cause less sleep disturbance and nightmares.
https://bnf.nice.org.uk/treatment-summaries/beta-adrenoceptor-blocking-drugs/

385 B – Atorvastatin

Avoid grapefruit juice as it is an enzyme inhibitor.
https://bnf.nice.org.uk/drugs/atorvastatin/

386 E – Metronidazole

Avoid alcohol due to risk of disulfiram like reaction.
https://bnf.nice.org.uk/drugs/metronidazole/
https://www.theindependentpharmacy.co.uk/bacterial-vaginosis-bv/
guides/metronidazole-alcohol

387 D – Carbimazole

Due to risk of idiosyncratic neutropenia.
https://bnf.nice.org.uk/drugs/carbimazole/

388 B - Advise Mr SA that combination NRT or varenicline have all been shown to be effective

All effective methods that can support patients to stop smoking.
https://cks.nice.org.uk/topics/smoking-cessation/

389 E - To provide the service, contractors must have a carbon monoxide (CO) monitor

https://psnc.org.uk/national-pharmacy-services/advanced-services/
smoking-cessation-service/

390 D - Lymecycline

Avoid lymecycline due to staining risk. It is contra-indicated in those under 8 years. (Deposition in growing bone and teeth, by binding to calcium, causes staining and occasionally dental hypoplasia).
https://bnf.nice.org.uk/drugs/lymecycline/

Case based discussion answers

391 Key areas to cover:

Review travel recommendations regarding vaccine/prevention based on location:

https://www.travelhealthpro.org.uk/

Give appropriate advice regarding travel, DEET spray, general health etc

Consider options if the patient was traveling with family? Is the patient pregnant or breastfeeding?

Any regular medication (if she is going for 6 months does she need to register as a temp patient whilst abroad?)

Review Maalof protect over the counter guidance if it is supplied from pharmacy *https://www.medicines.org.uk/emc/product/660/smpc*

392 Key areas to cover:

Consider all options e.g. NRT/varenicline/buprinoin etc.

https://cks.nice.org.uk/topics/smoking-cessation/

https://www.medicines.org.uk/emc/product/13451/smpc

Review various nicotine based products that are available to patient

https://bnf.nice.org.uk/drugs/nicotine/

Consider those options where patients are referred to community:

https://psnc.org.uk/national-pharmacy-services/advanced-services/smoking-cessation-service/

Can you signpost patient to services where they can have support with other peers?

393 Key areas to cover:

Discuss with the patient regarding compliance (first time taking medication, they may not understand the need for long term indication).

Consider possible drug options, e.g. aspirin, clopidogrel, atorvastatin, ramipril, GTN spray, bisoprolol and lansoprazole.

For each possible drug list indication, duration of treatment and whether routine monitoring is needed. Consider medicines management to support patient with new medication. Review NICE and BNF guidance re secondary prevention.

https://cks.nice.org.uk/topics/mi-secondary-prevention/

394 Consider:

What other medication may be co-prescribed?

Access local guidance for standard dosing

The standard prophylaxis dose is 3mg/kg

The standard treatment dose is 5mg/kg

Non-obese: Use actual body weight to determine the dose.

For obese patients: usually use ideal body weight. Gentamicin distributes poorly into adipose tissue. Patients who are obese should receive a relatively lower dose of gentamicin.

Dosing interval is usually based on renal function (e.g. the lower the renal function, the more frequent the interval).

Take pre dose levels up to one hour before the second dose is given.

Patients >65 years old, or with abnormal renal function or poor urine output - the pre dose gentamicin level must be ≤1mg/litre before any further dose is given (Anything above is classed as high).

For patients with normal and stable renal function check pre dose level twice weekly.

Also consider side effects.

Example of local guidance:

https://www.ruh.nhs.uk/For_Clinicians/departments_ruh/Pathology/documents/ haematology/Dosing_of_Gentamicin_Vancomycin_and_Teicoplanin.pdf
https://bnf.nice.org.uk/treatment-summaries/aminoglycosides/
https://bnf.nice.org.uk/drugs/gentamicin/#indications-and-dose

395 Consider:

Compliance: how many days have been missed, is there any chance of pregnancy, when was their last menses, are their menses regular, have they experienced irregular bleeding and do they have a regular partner? When did UPSI take place? What is the number of missed pills and the timing of pills (e.g. after her break of pills)? Yasmin is usually taken over three weeks and then a break, however in some cases patients may take them back to back. Confirm their duration and dose.

If the emergency pill applied, consider all 3 options for patient: copper coil, ellaOne and Levonelle.

Consider the risks vs the benefits of all treatments.

Consider the cost, efficacy, timing of UPSI and licensing.

Is the patient breastfeeding?

Counsel patient on the side effects and when to take another dose.

Consider the patient parameters, e.g. raised BMI? Antiepileptic medication?

396 Consider:

For learning purposes, consider the different types of women who will take/use HRT, e.g. hysterectomy, menopausal, peri-menopausal etc.

Consider the different types of options: oestrogen only, sequential combined and continuous combined.

Consider the routes available: topical, oral, patches, local acting etc.

When is it appropriate to prescribe certain HRT?

When is it appropriate to stop HRT?

Any modifiable lifestyle factors to improve HRT symptoms?

Any contraindications?

Consider the risks vs benefits of treatment with HRT.

At the annual review, reinforce lifestyle measures and check efficacy, side-effects, ensure correct dose, optimal route of delivery and compliance. Also check the risks vs benefits of continuing. The risk of breast cancer rises with long-term use. Check BP, encourage engagement with national screening programmes (breast/bowel/cervical) as appropriate.

Assess osteoporosis risk & consider the need for investigation/monitoring.

Enquire about symptoms of urogenital atrophy.

Review local guidance if possible.

https://cks.nice.org.uk/topics/menopause/prescribing-information/hormone-replacement-therapy-hrt

397 Consider:

Allergies, past medical history (e.g. history of tonsillitis) and general health.

Any medication that may cause a sore throat (in which a sore throat is a red flag).

Any viral symptoms

Examination: tonsils inflamed? What is the colour of the tonsils and is there any pus?

Does the patient have a cough, any rigours or a temperature?

Check physical observations, e.g. pulse, resp rate and any shortness of breath.

Consider red flags, e.g. quinsy or cancer.

Consider when to manage OTC, when to refer to GP / 111.

What options are available OTC.

Safety netting to patients.

398 Consider:

POM to P guidance

Can pharmacists make the diagnosis of migraine in order for OTC sale?

When is sumatriptan contraindicated?

Who is eligible (inclusion criteria), who is not eligible (exclusion criteria) – consider the license.

Consider the symptoms of a migraine which make them different to other headaches.

What other medication options or non pharmacological options are available to patients who suffer with migraines?

399 Consider:

Have live lice been seen on Miss KL? Is there an outbreak in school/nursery? Any siblings?

Any medical history, e.g. eczema, asthma or allergies.

Consider types of treatments available.

Consider duration of action.

Wet combing method?

https://cks.nice.org.uk/topics/head-lice/management/management/

400 Consider:

Indication for this medication? For example, usually symptomatic anaemia associated with chronic renal failure (CRF) in patients on dialysis.

Dose can be S/C or IV.

Based on weight.

Consider MHRA alerts, e.g. very rare risk of severe cutaneous adverse reactions.

Monitoring includes BP, reticulocyte counts, Hb and electroltes.

Correct iron/folate deficiency that contribute to anaemia of CRF before initiation, e.g. supplemental iron.

Index